Children
With
Special
Health Care
Needs

Nutrition
Care
Handbook

Editor: **Betty L. Lucas, MPH, RD**

Assistant Editors: **Sharon A. Feucht, MA, RD, and Lynn E. Grieger, RD, CDE**

Pediatric Nutrition Practice Group and
Dietetics in Developmental and Psychiatric Disorders

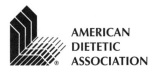

AMERICAN
DIETETIC
ASSOCIATION

10 9 8 7 6 5 4 3 2 1

Library of Congress Cataloging-in-Publication Data

Children with special health care needs : nutrition care handbook / Betty L. Lucas, Sharon A. Feucht, and Lynn E. Grieger, editors; Pediatric Nutrition Practice Group and Dietetics in Developmental and Psychiatric Disorders, American Dietetic Association.—1st ed.
    p. ; cm.
  Includes bibliographical references and index.
  ISBN 0–88091-346–0
1. Nutrition disorders in children—Handbooks, manuals, etc. 2. Children—Nutrition—Handbooks, manuals, etc. 3. Diet therapy for children—Handbooks, manuals, etc. 4. Children—Diseases—Nutritional aspects—Handbooks, manuals, etc.
  [DNLM: 1. Child Nutrition Disorders—diet therapy—Handbooks. 2. Nutrition Therapy—methods—Child—Handbooks. 3. Child Health Services—Handbooks. 4. Child, Exceptional—Handbooks. 5. Disabled Children—Handbooks. WS 39 C5367 2004] I. Lucas, Betty L. II. Feucht, Sharon A. III. Grieger, Lynn. IV. American Dietetic Association. Pediatric Nutrition Practice Group. V. American Dietetic Association. Dietetics in Developmental and Psychiatric Disorders Dietetic Practice Group.
RJ206.C5188 2004
613.2'083—dc22

2004011505

Contents

Chapter 3: Feeding and Eating   59

Chapter 4: Non-oral Enteral Feeding   87

Chapter 5: Fluid and Bowel Problems   103

Chapter 6: Community Services and Programs   119

Acknowledgments

This handbook is a revision of *Children with Special Health Care Needs: A Community Nutrition Pocket Guide,* which was originally published in 1997. The original publication was developed and supported by two dietetic practice groups of the American Dietetic Association—Dietetics in Developmental and Psychiatric Disorders (DDPD) and the Pediatric Nutrition Practice Group (PNPG). The pocket guide became reality only when Ross Products Division, Abbott Laboratories, provided generous support for publication and printing.

We wish to acknowledge the time and expertise of the original six authors (Janet Isaacs, Josephine Cialone, Janet Willis, Molly Holland, Patricia Murray, and Maria Nardella), who also contributed to this edition. Together they represent many decades of providing leadership and service to children with special health care needs and their families.

We appreciate the continued support of DDPD and PNPG in this revised publication, especially to the editorial leadership provided by Betty Lucas, editor, and Sharon Feucht and Lynn Grieger, assistant editors. We also acknowledge the contributions of the reviewers, many of them representing PNPG and DDPD.

Contributors

Editor

Betty L. Lucas, MPH, RD
Center on Human Development and Disability
University of Washington
Seattle, WA

Assistant Editors

Sharon A. Feucht, MA, RD
Center on Human Development and Disability
University of Washington
Seattle, WA

Lynn E. Grieger, RD, CDE
Professional Nutrition Services
Arlington, VT

Authors

Josephine A. Cialone, MS, RD
Nutrition Services Branch
North Carolina Division of Public Health
Raleigh, NC

Molly Holland, MPH, RD
Children with Special Health Needs
Vermont Department of Health
Burlington, VT

Janet Sugarman Isaacs, PhD, RD
Genetics and Metabolism Division
Children's National Medical Center
Washington, DC

Patricia Murray, MEd, RD
Department of Health and Human Services
Special Medical Services
Concord, NH

Maria T. Nardella, MA, RD
Children with Special Health Care Needs Program
Washington State Department of Health
Olympia, WA

Aaron Owens-Kuehner, MS, RD
Providence Children's Center
Everett, WA

Janet Horsley Willis, MPH, RD
Virginia LEND Program
Virginia Commonwealth University
Richmond, VA

Reviewers

Anne Bradford Harris, PhD, MPH, RD
Los Angeles, CA

Digna I. Cassens, MHA, RD
La Habra Heights, CA

Harriet H. Cloud, MS, RD, FADA
Birmingham, AL

Barbara Emison Gaffield, MS, RD
Williamsburg, VA

Sister Mary Catherine Faller, MS, RD
Cincinnati, OH

Joan E. Guthrie Medlen, RD
Portland, OR

Pamela S. Leeman, RD
Fayetteville, NC

Kim M. Nowak-Cooperman, MS, RD
Seattle, WA

Beth N. Ogata, MS, RD
Bellevue, WA

Diana C. Pantalos, MS, RD
Louisville, KY

Janelle D. Peterson, RD
Minneapolis, MN

Anita C. Rickard, RD, MA
Louisville, KY

Lea A. Theriot, MS, RD
Baton Rouge, LA

Cynthia L. Van Riper, MS, RD
Omaha, NE

Lee Shelly Wallace, MS, RD, FADA
Chattanooga, TN

Letitia B. Warren, RD
Allen Park, MI

Beth A. Zupec-Kania, RD
Elm Grove, WI

Foreword

Thirty six years ago, a number of dietitians accepted positions in a new program sponsored by the Maternal and Child Health Bureau at 21 different universities throughout the United States. Those programs were called University Affiliated Facilities, and their purpose was to provide leadership education for graduate students in nutrition and many other disciplines intending to work with children with developmental disabilities. Dietitians who completed these training programs demonstrated their leadership in the American Dietetic Association (ADA) by initiating the organization of two practice groups, Dietetics in Developmental and Psychiatric Disorders (DDPD) and the Pediatric Nutrition Practice Group (PNPG). Members of these two practice groups have collaborated in many ways, such as providing programs for the annual meeting of ADA, working together on legislative issues and position papers, and coauthoring publications.

This publication, *Children with Special Health Care Needs: Nutrition Care Handbook,* represents one of their collaborative efforts. This edition meets an important need as a handbook for many dietitians who serve an ever-increasing number of children with special health care needs such as developmental disabilities, mental retardation, birth defects, low birth weight, metabolic disorders, and other disorders. In the past, these children were often institutionalized, but because policies emphasizing inclusion have emerged in the last three decades, they are now seen in all areas of community health services, where they encounter and need the services of dietitians. It is estimated that the total number of adults and children with developmental disabilities is between 3 million and 7 million. Surveys indicate that approximately 800,000 children through 5 years of age have disabilities making them eligible for Early Intervention Services where nutrition is a designated fundable service. Surveys of these children found that approximately 50% have health problems placing them at nutritional risk. It was therefore obvious that this handbook would be a natural project for PNPG and DDPD, providing a resource for those practitioners monitoring the nutrition care of children with special health care needs.

I congratulate Betty Lucas, editor, Sharon Feucht and Lynn Grieger, assistant editors, and the authors, Janet Willis, Josephine Cialone, Maria Nardella, Janet Isaacs, Molly Holland, Patricia Murray, and Aaron Owens-Kuehner, for writing this very informative and useful nutrition handbook. Many dietitians will use it in providing and monitoring the nutrition care of the child with special health care needs.

Harriet Holt Cloud, MS, RD, FADA
Chair, Pediatric Nutrition Practice Group

Introduction

Children With Special Health Care Needs

Children with special health care needs (CSHCN) refers to children with a broad range of chronic illnesses and conditions who require health and related services beyond basic, routine care. Intervention generally means a range of medical, therapy, educational, financial, and family support services. CSHCN includes children with birth defects, neurological consequences of premature birth, genetic syndromes, sequelae of infection such as meningitis, and consequences of perinatal drug exposure. Also included in the definition of CSHCN are those "at risk" for chronic physical, developmental, and behavior conditions, such as children with very low birth weight, metabolic disorders, extreme poverty, or environmental exposure such as second-hand smoke or exposure to lead.

The number of CSHCN is increasing, due in part to advances in perinatal medicine, increased survival of premature infants, and early identification and treatment of many disorders. Compared with the past, when institutional care was more common, CSHCN today live with their families and receive medical care, education, and other resources in their communities. Current federal and state programs recommend that all services for CSHCN be coordinated, comprehensive, community-based, family-centered, and culturally competent.

Children with special health care needs are similar to children without special health care needs. They all require good nutrition to grow and develop. As a group, however, CSHCN have more frequent problems that may alter their growth, diet, feeding and eating behaviors, and bowel and fluid management. When these problems are not adequately addressed, the child may experience more infections and illness, fewer days in school or therapy, and greater health care costs for the family. These feeding and nutrition-related problems are also more likely to be chronic over time. The most common problems are:

- Altered growth, ie, underweight, overweight, short stature
- Inadequate energy and nutrient intake to support growth and health
- Feeding problems related to oral-motor and/or behavioral difficulties
- Medication-nutrient interactions
- Need for enteral (tube) feeding

- Chronic constipation or diarrhea
- Use of alternative or complementary therapies or products

Purpose of the Handbook

The purpose of the Handbook is to provide a quick reference for those monitoring the nutrition care of CSHCN. It is designed for readers who

- See a small number of children with special health care needs in their practice
- Are responding to a changing health care environment in which more children with chronic conditions are served in community settings
- Are receiving referrals for more children with complex nutrition and feeding problems
- May be more familiar with adult patients
- May usually work with typically developing children

After using the Handbook, the reader should be more comfortable working with these children and their families and be better able to communicate with the children's specialty service providers.

How to Use the Handbook

This Handbook is organized by common functional nutrition problems seen by dietetics professionals, primary care providers, and medical specialists. Although some problems are more often seen with specific diagnoses, there is much variation in children with the same diagnosis. The presenting growth concern, inadequate diet, or feeding difficulty is the referring problem that requires assessment and intervention. The Handbook includes information and guidance that health care providers are likely to need in serving CSHCN in outpatient and community settings. The authors' goal is to provide information to community colleagues working with families whose children have special health care needs to assist in screening and identification of nutrition problems, assessment, intervention, referral to specialty providers, and ongoing monitoring.

This Handbook is not comprehensive in addressing all of the complex nutrition problems of CSHCN seen in the community. Referral to specialty care and interdisciplinary teams is noted when appropriate. The Resource section includes a listing of more specific nutrition care books, manuals, Web sites, and other resources.

The chapters pertaining to growth, diet, feeding, and fluid and bowel management include a section related to healthy infants and children and then a section pertaining to alterations needed for CSHCN. The intervention section in every chapter is targeted toward CSHCN, with case examples of the assessment and intervention process at the end of each chapter. The last chapter on community services and programs outlines the variety of resources related to nutrition services within education programs, modified school meals, and sources of reimbursements for nutrition services and products. Each chapter also contains practical Clinical Tips that are based on the authors' experience.

It is anticipated that readers will use this Handbook as a resource when needed, rather than reading it through. Therefore, topics are cross-referenced between chapters, and the Glossary includes many conditions and terms used throughout the book.

Users of the Handbook

Many dietetics professionals may find this book helpful, including

- Dietitians who work in community hospitals with few pediatric patients
- Dietitians working in WIC or public health programs
- Dietitians with Head Start, Early Head Start, or school Child Nutrition Programs
- Dietitians consulting with early intervention programs serving children birth to age 3 years
- Dietitians working in home health agencies with few pediatric clients
- Dietitians working in community clinics serving high-risk or underserved populations
- Dietetics students in clinical and community pediatric rotations

Other health care providers will find this handbook useful, including primary care providers (pediatricians, family practitioners, pediatric nurse practitioners), public health nurses, school nurses, and health professionals working in early intervention programs, Head Start, Early Head Start, and similar programs serving CSHCN.

The overall nutrition goal for CSHCN is to ensure optimal nutritional status to support growth and development. This requires collaboration with families and coordination with other health and education professionals so that comprehensive and family-centered care is available to the child and family in their community. This Handbook provides readers a resource to make that goal happen.

Chapter 1

Growth

Josephine A. Cialone, MS, RD

The growth of infants and children is routinely monitored by a variety of health care providers. Most healthy children have steady growth rates, remaining within one or two growth channels over time. The ideal assessment of an individual child is based on a series of measurements gathered periodically in a consistent manner with reliable equipment.

Growth Charts

The Centers for Disease Control and Prevention (CDC) growth charts are used to assess physical measurements of stature or length and weight from infants, children, and adolescents up to 20 years of age, and head circumference measurements from infants and children up to 36 months of age. These charts are gender- and age-specific and can be used for most children with a birth weight more than 1,500 g. The CDC growth charts can be downloaded from the CDC Web site (http://www.cdc.gov/growthcharts).

The CDC growth charts allow for the following five growth indexes (1):

- Weight-for-age reflects body weight relative to age and is influenced by recent changes in health or nutritional status. Weight-for-age is not used to classify infants, children, and adolescents as underweight or overweight. However, weight-for-age is important in early infancy for monitoring weight and can also provide insights into changes in weight-for-length and body mass index (BMI)-for-age.
- Stature- or length-for-age describes linear growth relative to age. Stature- or length-for-age is used to define shortness or tallness.
- Weight-for-length reflects body weight relative to length and requires no knowledge of age. It is an indicator used to classify infants and young

children as overweight, underweight, or within normal limits for the length.

- BMI-for-age is an anthropometric index of weight and height combined with age. BMI-for-age is used to classify children and adolescents as underweight, overweight, at risk of overweight, or within normal limits for their age.
- Head circumference–for-age can be assessed up to 36 months of age. Head circumference is a critical growth parameter during infancy because these measurements reflect brain size. Head circumference–for-age can also identify possible abnormalities such as hydrocephalus.

When assessing weight and length of a premature infant, measures should be plotted based on adjusted/corrected age rather than actual age. To calculate adjusted/corrected age, subtract the number of weeks the infant was born prematurely from the current age of the infant. For example, a 5-month-old infant born prematurely at 32 weeks' gestation (8 weeks early) is 3 months adjusted/corrected age. The practice of using adjusted/corrected age when assessing a premature infant should continue until age 24 to 36 months, using the CDC growth charts for birth to 36 months.

Accurate assessment of growth depends on reliable measurements. Errors in measurements include the following:

- Using inappropriate technique
- Equipment inaccuracies and lack of calibration
- Inconsistency of measuring infant or child with clothing or shoes
- Measuring an infant or child with braces or casts
- Rounding errors from pounds/ounces, kilograms/grams, or inches/centimeters

Using the CDC Growth Charts to Assess Infants and Children

Table 1.1 summarizes the growth indexes that can be derived from the CDC growth charts (1).

The nutritional status indicators of the CDC growth charts include overweight, at risk of overweight, underweight, and short stature. Percentiles are used to rank an individual's measurement on a growth chart and indicate where that measurement fits in relation to the reference population. Table 1.2 summarizes ways the CDC growth charts can be used to determine indicators of nutritional status (1).

Other indicators can be derived from the CDC growth charts to express the status of an infant or child's growth. These indicators include the following:

- Weight-age equivalent: Age at which current weight would fall at the 50th percentile on the weight-for-age chart. (See Figure 1.1 for example of determining weight-age.)
- Height-age equivalent: Age at which current length or stature would fall at the 50th percentile on the height-for-age or length-for-age chart (See Figure 1.1 for example of determining height-age.)
- Ideal body weight for length or height: Weight at the 50th percentile for height-age.
- Percent ideal body weight: Current weight/weight at the 50th percentile for current length or height × 100. (Table 1.3 [2] lists the interpretation of the percent ideal body weight for children.)

No single indicator should be used to assess a child's nutritional status. Growth and weight gain of children with special health care needs are often affected by other factors related to their condition. Box 1.1 summarizes factors that may affect a child's growth and weight gain (3).

Table 1.1
Anthropometric Indexes of Growth From the CDC Growth Charts

Indexes	Information Derived	Conditions
Weight	• Weight percentile for chronological age • Weight percentile for age corrected for prematurity • Weight-age equivalent • Ideal body weight	• Underweight • Overweight • Obesity • Failure to thrive • Inadequate weight gain
Height/stature/length	• Length percentile for age • Length percentile for age corrected for prematurity • Height percentile for age • Height-age equivalent	• Short stature • Growth stunting
Head circumference	Head circumference percentile for age	• Microcephaly • Macrocephaly
Weight-for-length or BMI-for-age	Proportional percentile	• Underweight • Overweight • Obesity • Failure to thrive

Abbreviations: BMI, body mass index; CDC, Centers for Disease Control and Prevention.
Source: Data are from reference 1.

Table 1.2
Nutritional Status Indicators Using the CDC Growth Charts

Anthropometric Index	Percentile Cut-Off Value	Nutritional Status Indicator	Interpretation for Child With Special Health Care Needs*
BMI-for-age Weight-for-length/stature	> 95th	Overweight	• Common in Down syndrome or conditions that cause skeletal deformities such as spina bifida, scoliosis
BMI-for-age	> 85th and < 95th	At risk of overweight	• Common in conditions that limit ambulatory abilities
BMI-for-age Weight-for-length	< 5th	Underweight	• Common in conditions that limit muscle mass such as spastic quadriplegia cerebral palsy • Common in feeding disorders • Common in conditions that affect absorption and metabolism
Stature/length-for-age	< 5th	Short stature	• May be related to prenatal factor or genetic disorder • Usually seen in neurologic disorders with microcephaly
	> 95th	Tall for age	• Unusual, but characteristic of rare genetic disorders
Head circumference–for-age	< 5th > 95th	Microcephaly Macrocephaly	• Developmental problems

Abbreviations: BMI, body mass index; CDC, Centers for Disease Control and Prevention.
*Interpretation related to children with special health care needs is based on clinical practice.
Source: Data are from reference 1.

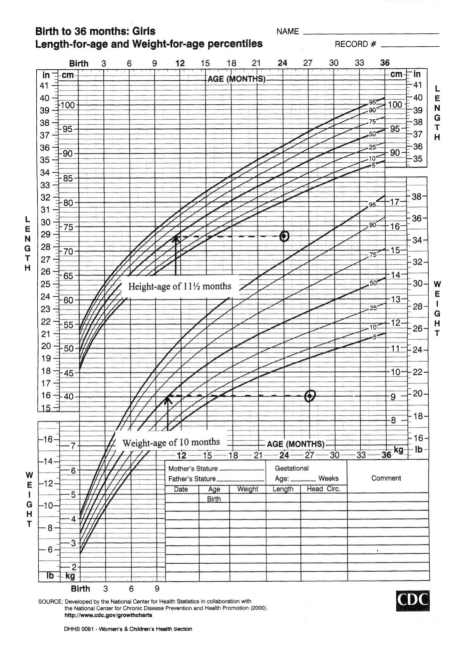

Figure 1.1 Determining weight-age and height-age equivalents.

Table 1.3
Interpretation of Percent Ideal Body Weight for Children

Percent Ideal Weight	Interpretation
> 110%	Overweight
90% to 110%	Normal
81% to 90%	Mild malnutrition
70% to 80%	Moderate malnutrition
< 70%	Severe malnutrition

Source: Data are from reference 2.

Clinical Tips

- Recumbent length and standing height (stature) are both appropriate for children in the age range of 24 to 36 months, but the appropriate CDC growth chart must be used based on the measurement method used.
- Use the sex-specific CDC growth chart for ages birth to 36 months when assessing recumbent length and the sex-specific CDC growth chart for ages 2 to 20 years when assessing standing height.
- Weight changes can occur more rapidly than changes in stature. Therefore, weight is a more sensitive indicator of current health and recent dietary intake than stature.
- Body mass index (BMI) is a measure of an individual's adiposity. BMI is the ratio of weight in kilograms to stature in meters squared (kg/m^2). Unlike adults, a child's BMI cannot be assessed independent of age. BMI may be affected if a child has hypertonia or hypotonia.

Incremental Weight Gain and Linear Growth

Assessment and interpretation of growth of children with special health care needs are different from assessment and interpretation of growth of typically developing children. The CDC growth charts do not account for growth expectations influenced by chronic disease or disability. A child's growth must be assessed within the context of medical status and genetic condition. Additional assessment of body composition may be recommended and the adequacy of dietary intake must be determined.

Incremental weight gain and linear growth can be used to assess progress toward expected growth in children with special health care needs. The expected mean daily weight gain for infants and toddlers is shown in Table 1.4 (4). The mean daily growth velocity for linear growth and weight gain for infants and toddlers is shown in Table 1.5 (4).

Box 1.1   Factors Affecting Children's Growth

Nutrition
- Nutritional adequacy of the infant or child's dietary intake, including amount consumed and feeding patterns.

Genetics
- Parental height and other genetic body composition factors.
- Family history of and existing medical condition(s) that affect the home environment, such as mental illness or retardation.

Psychosocial
- The home environment, family economic situation, and other factors that affect access to food, including customs and cultural practices that affect shopping, preparation, and provision of food for the child.
- A child's hunger and satiety cues and the family's ability to respond to appetite.

Medical
- Prenatal conditions such as alcohol or drug use, exposure to viral infection, and prenatal weight gain.
- Birth factors such as birth weight, head circumference, prematurity, initial feeding method (eg, tube, bottle, breast), lung disease, malabsorption, and family home adjustment after extended hospitalization or with chronic medical condition.
- Frequency and severity of acute illness and need for prescribed medications.

Diagnosis
- Chromosomal abnormalities are associated with growth patterns that differ from those of normal children.
- In children with metabolic disorders, affected metabolic pathways involved in producing energy or building body tissue may be altered.
- Children who are nonambulatory due to neurological conditions may not grow normally, possibly due to a lack of weight-bearing activities that normally provide physical stress on the long bones of the leg required to stimulate bone growth.
- Children with neurological conditions affecting ambulation may also have problems with feeding.

Source: Data are from reference 3.

Table 1.4
Expected Daily Weight Gain for Infants and Toddlers*

Age, mo	Mean Daily Weight Gain, oz (g)
Birth to 3	1.00 (28.2)
3 to 6	0.61 (16.8)
6 to 12	0.40 (11.3)
12 to 18	0.30 (8.5)
18 to 24	0.25 (7.0)

*Derived from incremental weight gain at 50th percentile.
Source: Data are from reference 4.

Table 1.5
Expected Daily Length Gain for Infants and Toddlers*

Age, mo	Mean Daily Length Gain, mm
Birth to 2	1.06
2 to 6	0.77
6 to 12	0.47
12 to 18	0.35
18 to 24	0.30

*Derived from incremental length gain at 50th percentile.
Source: Data are from reference 4.

Skinfold Thickness and Arm Circumference

Growth assessment is clarified by a measure of body composition. The rationale is that muscle (as part of the lean body mass) weighs more than other body components and is greatly affected by the central nervous system (CNS). Many children with special health care needs have conditions that reduce muscle mass. These children may appear thin, but this appearance is not necessarily the result of low body fat. Skinfold thickness and arm circumference can provide a more comprehensive picture of the child's nutritional status (5). Low muscle mass may be affected by many different factors in addition to nutritional status.

Arm circumference and skinfold thickness should be measured by a trained clinician to ensure accuracy. Arm circumference and skinfold measurements can be used in conjunction with other anthropometric data to gain insights when interpreting the child's weight status and determining trends in overnutrition or undernutrition over time (6). Table 1.6 describes the use of skinfold thickness and arm circumference measures and their nutritional implications.

Head Circumference

Deviations from the norm in head circumference measurements are common in children with special health care needs. The majority of these deviations are related to disease, genetic abnormalities, or prenatal nutrition, rather than to current nutritional status. Measurement of head circumference in all children is recommended. These measures can be assessed using the CDC growth charts for children younger than 3 years of age; the Nellhaus chart can be used to assess

Table 1.6
Use of Skinfold Thickness and Arm Circumference in Estimating Body Composition

Triceps Skinfold Percentile	Arm Circumference Percentile	Possible Interpretation*	Probable Appearance and Nutritional Implications*
< 5th	< 5th	• Low body fat and low muscle mass. • May be due to genetic or medical factors.	• Child appears thin; is underweight; increase calories.
< 5th	15th to 50th	• Low body fat with adequate muscle mass. • Consider recent illness, weight loss, or inadequate nutrition in the past.	• Child appears thin; is underfat; increase calories. • Body fat should increase to match or exceed muscle mass.
15th to 50th	< 5th	• Adequate body fat with low muscle mass. • Possible central nervous system origin.	• Child appears thin; is not underweight. • Assess activity level.
15th to 50th	50th to 85th	• Larger muscle mass than fat stores. • Possibly from extensive use of upper body, eg, use of wheelchair or walker.	• Child appears large; is not overweight. • Assess activity level.

*Interpretation related to children with special health care needs is based on clinical practice.

older children (7). Head circumference percentile is generally closely aligned with the percentile for linear growth. The interpretation of head circumference measures using charts is reviewed in Table 1.7.

Bone Age/Skeletal Age

Skeletal maturation occurs within a predictable sequence of events. Fusion of the epiphysis and the appearance of ossification centers occur in a predictable order. Bone or skeletal age is usually measured by an x-ray of the hand and wrist. Bone age is often used to evaluate a child whose linear growth is proceeding at an unusual rate. Delayed or accelerated bone growth can be used for diagnosis of certain syndromes or to estimate the potential for catch-up growth.

Special Interpretations from CDC Growth Charts

There can be both nutritional and non-nutritional reasons for different growth patterns. It is important to limit nutrition recommendations to those circumstances in which nutritional factors are contributory and to set realistic growth expectations for the individual child.

Most children with special health care needs have diagnoses for which there are no standardized growth charts. Children with special health care needs were not included in the reference population used as the basis for the CDC growth charts. Therefore, the CDC growth charts should be used with careful interpretation. The most accurate assessment can be achieved by monitoring growth and

Table 1.7
Head Circumference and Growth Assessment

Head Circumference	Interpretation*
< 5th percentile in child younger than 3 y who was not born prematurely	Microcephaly • Will generally match height percentile • May result from small-for-gestational age or prenatal factor
< 2nd percentile in child older than 3 y	Microcephaly • Will generally match height percentile
Decrease in percentile over time in infancy	• Requires neurological evaluation • Possible inadequate brain growth
Increase in percentile over time in infancy	• Requires neurological evaluation • Hydrocephalus

*Interpretation related to children with special health care needs is based on clinical practice.

weight gain over time. Goals for growth and weight gain can only be determined with consideration of other parameters of nutrition assessment such as dietary intake, biochemical values, and medical and psychosocial factors.

Collecting anthropometric measurements on children older than 3 years of age who cannot stand can sometimes be difficult. Using the same technique, especially for stature, is important each time data is collected at subsequent visits. Alternative methods to obtain weight and stature measurements in children who cannot stand are outlined in Table 1.8.

Specialized Growth Charts

The CDC growth charts are appropriate for assessing low-birth-weight infants (1,501 to 2,500 g) because they are included in the reference population for these charts. The Infant Health and Developmental Program (IHDP) growth charts can be used for very-low-birth-weight infants (≤ 1,500 g) after discharge (8).

Several specialized charts are available for assessing growth of infants and children with certain conditions and syndromes. These include achondroplasia, spastic quadriplegia cerebral palsy, Down syndrome, Marfan syndrome, Noonan syndrome, Prader-Willi syndrome, spina bifida, Turner syndrome, and Williams syndrome. There are some limitations to the specialized charts because they were developed based on a limited sample size and may not reflect current standards of nutrition treatment. In most cases, these specialty charts do not include all growth parameters. These charts should be viewed as additional indexes to be used along with the CDC growth charts. Samples of specialty

Table 1.8
Alternative Anthropometric Measures for Children Who Cannot Stand

Measure	Accommodation
Weight of a child unable to stand	• Use standard procedure for weighing infants • Weigh parent and child; subtract parent's weight • Use chair scale, bed scale, or wheelchair scale, if available
Stature of a child unable to stand (6)	• Use recumbent length • Use crown-rump length • Use sitting height • Use lower leg length* • Use arm span*

*Requires trained clinician to perform technique.

growth charts are available in the *Pediatric Manual of Clinical Nutrition,* 2nd edition (9–14).

Clinical Tips

- Providers who do not routinely collect skinfold measurements should not attempt to gather and assess these measures because the rate of error is too great.
- A bone-age study can help predict a successful outcome for starting a nutrition intervention. If a child with failure to thrive, low weight-for-age, and low length/stature-for-age is found to have a delayed bone-age, catch-up growth can likely be achieved with aggressive nutrition support. If a delayed bone-age is noted along with a renal or endocrine disorder, the potential for catch-up is not as directly related to nutrition.
- Some families consider weight gain to be an index of health for their premature infant. Practitioners need to be sensitive to the family's anxiety and concern when interpreting slow growth in an infant who may have special needs.
- Muscular children may be incorrectly evaluated as overweight or obese when using only anthropometric measures plotted on a CDC growth chart. Skinfold thickness and arm circumference data can delineate those who have a high muscle mass and those who are truly overweight or obese.
- Children with low muscle mass whose weight-for-length or BMI-for-age are in the lower percentiles may be considered underweight until their skinfold measures determine that they in fact have adequate fat stores. Such children often are picky eaters with small appetites and low intakes.
- Use ideal body weight (IBW) if previous growth measurements are not available. However, IBW assumes normal body composition and may not fit some children with neurologic disabilities who have low muscle mass.

Medications

A variety of medications used by children with special health care needs can directly or indirectly affect growth. For example, long-term use of corticosteroids may contribute to fluid retention, muscle wasting, and bone fragility. The result is reduced rates of linear growth and weight gain. Decreased nutrient intake may result from other medications that affect appetite or cause nausea, vomiting, or gastrointestinal distress. Reduced rates of growth and weight gain may be seen in this circumstance. See Chapter 2 for a more detailed discussion of this topic.

Supporting Optimal Growth

Nutritional approaches for improving growth rate in children with special health care needs are the same as for other children. Dietary assessment and intervention are discussed in Chapter 2. However, nutritional approaches may not be effective if a genetic or medical diagnosis that affects the growth pattern is present. In that situation, the intervention goal is to assure that undernutrition or malnutrition is not superimposed, because these would also limit growth. Table 1.9 outlines nutritional and non-nutritional factors to consider when assessing weight gain and linear growth.

When non-nutritional factors are determined to be responsible for inadequate growth, appropriate therapies, medical treatment, or resources should be provided. When genetics or particular syndromes determine the child's growth pattern, the family should be reassured that their child is attaining adequate growth. Support groups for families with children with the same condition may be beneficial. Periodic reassessment and monitoring should be scheduled.

Table 1.9
Factors in Assessing Abnormal Growth and Weight

Anthropometric Indexes	Non-nutritional Factor	Nutritional Factor
Short stature	• Genetic influences • Chronic illness • Diagnosis with associated short stature, eg, Down syndrome • Endocrine disorder	• Inadequate nutrient intake • Increased nutrient needs resulting from medical condition
Inadequate weight gain and/or underweight	• Oral-motor dysfunction • Malabsorption • Decreased appetite resulting from medications • Vomiting, severe reflux, diarrhea • Family disruption resulting from poor parenting skills, or drug or alcohol use • Inadequate financial resources to provide food	• Inadequate nutrient intake • Increased nutrient needs resulting from medical condition
Excessive weight gain and/or overweight	• Genetic syndromes • Skeletal anomalies • Nonambulatory status • Medication side effects	• Excessive energy intake • Decreased energy needs related to diagnosis

When nutritional factors are determined partially or primarily responsible for inadequate growth, specific interventions should be planned. Goals for achieving adequate energy and nutrient intake using appropriate feeding methods should be developed with family input. Refer to Chapters 2 and 3 for guidance in determining these goals.

Case Examples

Example 1

Patient
A nonambulatory 4-year-old boy with severe mental retardation.

Problem
The family has recently moved to the area and medical history and past anthropometric measurements are not available.

Findings
Mother reports that the child has always been small for age and underweight. She assists the child in transferring to a wheelchair, which he takes to preschool. Growth parameters are as follows:

- Height-for-age < 5th percentile
- Weight-for-age < 5th percentile
- BMI-for-age < 5th percentile
- Head circumference < 5th percentile

The child enjoys eating thickened or pureed foods and the family does not consider feeding a problem.

Recommendations

- Assist the family in locating specialty care providers and evaluation services.
- Obtain appropriate releases to obtain previous medical records to assess his growth pattern.
- Schedule a return visit to monitor and reassess growth, with the plan to review the child's medical history to determine if a nutrition care plan for both preschool and home can be developed.
- Possible goal: BMI-for-age at the 10th percentile.

Rationale

Although the child is at risk for undernutrition based on all growth parameters, insufficient evidence is available to complete the assessment. The child's poor linear growth status and microcephaly is likely due to the mental retardation, but appropriate nutrition intervention should support a BMI-for-age at the 10th percentile. Additional information about safely progressing textures must be obtained prior to developing a plan for nutrition intervention.

Example 2

Patient

An ambulatory 7-year-old girl with hemiplegic cerebral palsy.

Problem

The child's mother thinks that her daughter should be taller and encourages her to eat more than the child wants.

Findings

Growth parameters are as follows:

- Weight-for-age at 10th percentile
- Height-for-age < 5th percentile
- BMI-for-age at the 25th percentile
- Triceps skinfold at the 5th to 50th percentile
- Arm circumference at the 85th to 95th percentile
- Head circumference–for-age at the 25th percentile

The mother reports that the child eats small portions and does not have a good appetite. The clinic nurse is concerned that the child may not be receiving adequate nutrition at home. The dietary intake analysis documents that the child consumes adequate energy from a variety of foods with no inappropriate feeding practices.

Recommendations

- Assure mother that child's overall growth status is adequate.
- Monitor the child's growth over the next 6 months.

Rationale

While this child has short stature, her BMI-for-age, triceps skinfold, and arm circumference are within normal limits and indicate adequate nutrition.

Example 3

Patient
A 2-year-old girl with seizure disorder.

Problem
Early Intervention Program therapist has documented that this child is underweight and is recommending weight gain.

Findings
Growth parameters:

- Weight-for-age at the 5th percentile
- Length-for-age at the 5th percentile
- Weight-for-length at the 5th percentile
- Head circumference–for-age < 5th percentile

The parents express concern about their daughter's weight status but think that she is exhibiting typical "picky" eating for a child her age. The parents express apprehension about encouraging an increased rate of weight gain because they have tried a variety of supplements, but they have not been accepted by the child.

Recommendations

- Determine energy and nutrient intake and consider recommendations for modifications with family input.
- Refer for evaluation of possible feeding problems.
- Due to apprehensiveness of family to encourage weight gain, consider moderate increase in energy intake and set goals for small increments of weight gain.
- Monitor the child's growth, weight gain, and dietary intake over the next several months.

Rationale
The family's priorities for the child must be considered in developing the nutrition care plan. A more aggressive approach to weight gain may be accepted once a relationship with the family has been established and feeding problems have been ruled out.

Example 4

Patient
A low-birth-weight 7-month-old girl who was born at 32 weeks' gestation.

Problem
The infant is referred by Early Intervention due to concerns about weight gain and growth.

Findings
Growth parameters are as follows:

- Birth weight 1,750 g
- Weight-for-age < 5th percentile
- Length-for-age < 5th percentile
- Weight-for-length at the 5th percentile
- Head circumference–for age < 5th percentile

The mother reports that the infant's neonatal hospital course was unremarkable; she was discharged on 22-kcal-per-ounce premature formula and continues to receive that formula along with a limited amount of strained foods and rice cereal.

Recommendations
- Determine percentiles weight- and length-for-adjusted age.
- Determine rate of incremental weight gain and linear growth.
- Determine dietary intake and feeding development.
- Consider increased energy intake to support catch-up growth.

Rationale
The infant's weight-for-length indicates that the infant is lean and may benefit from an increased energy intake. Plotting weight- and length-for-adjusted age will provide information on expectation for catch-up growth. Analysis of the dietary intake will offer insights into the nutrient intake and appropriateness of sources of energy.

References

1. Centers for Disease Control and Prevention. Use and Interpretation of CDC Growth Charts. Available at: http://www.cdc.gov/nccdphp/dnpa/growthcharts/guide_intro.htm. Accessed January 6, 2004.

2. Nutrition assessment of infants and children. In: Nevin-Folino NF, ed. *Pediatric Manual of Clinical Dietetics*. 2nd ed. Chicago, Ill: American Dietetic Association; 2003:156–147.

3. Maternal and Child Health Bureau, Health Services and Resources Administration, Department of Health and Human Services. Growth Patterns of Children with Special Needs. Available at: http://depts.washington.edu/growth/cshcn/text/page2b.htm. Accessed January 6, 2004.

4. Appendix 21: growth velocity charts for gains in weight and length. In: Nevin-Folino NF, ed. *Pediatric Manual of Clinical Dietetics*. 2nd ed. Chicago, Ill: American Dietetic Association; 2003:775–776.

5. Zemel B, Stallings V. Energy requirements and nutritional assessment in developmental disabilities. In: Walker WA, Watkins JB, eds. *Nutrition in Pediatrics*. Hamilton, Ontario: BC Decker, Inc; 1996:169–177.

6. Feucht S. Assessment of growth: part 1, equipment, technique and growth charts. *Nutrition Focus*. 2000;15(2):1–8.

7. Nellhaus G. Composite international and interracial graphs. *Pediatrics*. 1968;41:106.

8. Appendix 20: IHDP growth percentiles. In: Nevin-Folino NF, ed. *Pediatric Manual of Clinical Dietetics*. 2nd ed. Chicago, Ill: American Dietetic Association; 2003:767–768, 771–772.

9. Appendix 23: Down syndrome. In: Nevin-Folino NF, ed. *Pediatric Manual of Clinical Dietetics*. 2nd ed. Chicago, Ill: American Dietetic Association; 2003:787–794.

10. Appendix 24: girls with Turner syndrome, physical growth 2 to 19 years. In: Nevin-Folino NF, ed. *Pediatric Manual of Clinical Dietetics*. 2nd ed. Chicago, Ill: American Dietetic Association; 2003:795.

11. Appendix 25: cerebral palsy (spastic quadriplegic). In: Nevin-Folino NF, ed. *Pediatric Manual of Clinical Dietetics*. 2nd ed. Chicago, Ill: American Dietetic Association; 2003:796–801.

12. Appendix 26: Prader-Willi syndrome. In: Nevin-Folino NF, ed. *Pediatric Manual of Clinical Dietetics*. 2nd ed. Chicago, Ill: American Dietetic Association; 2003:802–803.

13. Appendix 27: achondroplasia. In: Nevin-Folino NF, ed. *Pediatric Manual of Clinical Dietetics*. 2nd ed. Chicago, Ill: American Dietetic Association; 2003:804–808.

14. Appendix 28: Noonan syndrome. In: Nevin-Folino NF, ed. *Pediatric Manual of Clinical Dietetics*. 2nd ed. Chicago, Ill: American Dietetic Association; 2003:809–810.

Chapter 2

Diet and Nutrition

Molly Holland, MPH, RD, and Patricia Murray, MEd, RD

Nutrition Screening

The process of screening for nutrition and feeding issues is an important function of any health care team. Many screening instruments have been developed for identification of nutrition concerns. Two that are commonly used include the "PEACH" questionnaire (1) and "A look at nutrition" (2). Ideally, a screening instrument is simple to administer and identifies nutrition and feeding issues that the parents/caregivers are having with their child. Because socioeconomic circumstances can affect the child's dietary intake and health, these areas should also be assessed. Table 2.1 lists the major areas to address in a screening tool used to identify nutrition and feeding concerns (3).

Dietary Assessment

The process of assessing the intake of a child with special health care needs is the same as assessing any other child. However there often are additional areas to review. Table 2.2 identifies information that should be obtained in a general pediatric dietary assessment and includes special considerations that should be noted when completing a dietary assessment for a child with special health care needs (3). (Note: This chapter focuses on information related to dietary assessment of nutrients whereas Chapter 5 focuses on assessment of dietary fiber and fluid needs.)

Chronic Health Conditions and Nutrition-Related Concerns

The underlying medical condition that the child with special health care needs has can have a direct (primary) or indirect (secondary) effect on the child's overall growth and development. Table 2.3 can be used as a guide when assessing

Table 2.1

Areas of Focus for Screening for Nutrition and Feeding Issues in Children

Area of Focus	Nutritional Risk Factors: Refer if . . .
Concerns about food intake, feeding, and nutrition	Inadequate or inappropriate dietary intake for >3 days
Child's typical feeding pattern (types of foods eaten and how often)	Alternative or special diet (vegan, multiple food allergies, etc) Consumes only liquids, pureed foods, or ground foods after age 2 years Pica (intake of nonfood items)
Use of nutritional supplements	Used on a regular basis for supplementation of the diet
Use of vitamin/mineral supplements	Use of supplements exceeding 100% DRIs/ULs without physician approval
Use of complementary/alternative nutritional therapies	Intentional omission of a food group (such as milk, dairy) Unproven herbal supplementation
Adequacy of food resources and participation in eligible food and nutrition programs	Inadequate food supply Financial difficulties

Abbreviations: DRI, dietary reference intake; UL, tolerable upper intake level.
Source: Data are from reference 3.

Clinical Tip

Although food diaries may be difficult for parents and caregivers to complete, they can provide the dietetics professional with a wealth of information. Food diaries should include the following information: time and length of meal, location, food offered, food consumed, food lost from mouth, and use of medications or supplements. It is also helpful to describe if the day recorded was "typical" or unusual in some way, the child's general health, and physical activities during the day. Because caregivers may over- or underreport, the dietetics professional should review the food diary and verify the portions with measuring cups, spoons, bottles, and food models. The most common errors are omitting liquids and small snacks between scheduled meal times. Having the parent/caregiver relate eating with the day's activities is a good way to help them remember small snacks and fluids consumed. If the child is also experiencing issues with vomiting or constipation, this information can be recorded in the food diary.

Table 2.2
Dietary Assessment

Information to Obtain for All Pediatric Clients	Special Considerations for Children with Special Needs
Food intake	
Type, brand name, and amount of food, beverages, or formula actually consumed at a meal or snack	Child may lose food from mouth due to oral-motor feeding problems or vomiting; may be helpful to observe a meal or snack.
Preparation methods for foods and formula	Recipes may be modified by addition of fat, sugars, or protein. Request exact recipe for formula, including ingredients, amounts, preparation methods and storage.
Favorite foods, food dislikes, food jags, food allergies, or intolerances	Determine how eating patterns and intake are altered when the child is ill or when there is a change in the medical condition or medication (eg, child refuses to eat or reduced fluid intake).
Frequency, length, and location of meals and snacks	Obtain food diaries (both weekdays and weekend); determine how many people feed the child throughout the day; observe an actual meal or snack.
Child's independence in obtaining food	If the child is dependent on others to be fed, determine whether the feeders can identify hunger and fullness.
Current and past use of nutrition supplements or special diets	May indicate nutritional risk or a history of nutritional risk from a medical condition.
Other factors that influence intake	
Cultural or ethnic family eating practices	Determine family's beliefs and values regarding feeding a child with a disability or special health care needs.
Use of complementary/alternative nutrition therapies	Determine if and how this affects the child's food intake; determine exact amounts of supplements and cost.
Activity level or ambulation	Affects energy needs if child is overactive or limited in mobility.
Pertinent eating/feeding history	Determine whether feeding history correlates with the child's advancement in other areas of development.

(continued)

Table 2.2   (*continued*)

Information to Obtain for All Pediatric Clients	Special Considerations for Children with Special Needs
Parent's perception of the role of nutrition/feeding practices as they relate to the child's health condition	Helps determine the degree of knowledge and/or stress parents/caregivers may be experiencing with their children's eating/feeding or growth.
Caregiver's ability to recognize hunger and satiety cues	Lack of awareness may alter the child's intake (either feeding more or less than required).
Other programs or therapies that may be providing food as a reward/therapy	If close to mealtimes, may affect a child's intake.

Source: Data are from reference 3.

children with a known diagnosis (4,5). Some children may not exhibit all the identified risk factors at the time of the assessment, but the problem may arise at a later date.

Dietary Intake

Dietary assessment involves determining the nutrient intake of the child and comparing this intake to standards. Tables 2.4, 2.5, and 2.6 present commonly accepted guidelines for determining the dietary intake of all infants and children (6,7).

Clinical Tips

- A good rule for recommended serving sizes is 1 Tbsp of each of the food groups per age, per meal.
- The question of when and how much juice to introduce to infant diets is an ongoing discussion because a high intake of juice early in life has been associated with dental caries and reduced intake of other nutrients (protein, fat, iron, etc) (8). The American Academy of Pediatrics (AAP) recommends that juices be provided to infants 6 months of age or older or when they can drink from a cup. Infants should not be put to bed with a bottle. AAP also recommends no more than 4 to 6 oz of juice per day as part of a meal or snack for children ages 1 to 6. For older children and adolescents ages 7 to 18 years, the AAP recommends the maximum of 8 to 12 oz of juice per day (8).
- Infants and children who have a family history of allergies may be advised by their pediatrician to avoid foods commonly associated with severe allergic reactions. See Food Allergy/Intolerances section of this chapter for more information.

(*continued on page 29*)

Table 2.3
Selected Syndromes and Developmental Disabilities: Frequently Reported Nutrition Problems and Factors Contributing to Nutritional Risk

Syndrome/ Disability	Altered Growth, Underweight, Obesity	Altered Energy Needs	Constipation or Diarrhea	Feeding Problems	Other
Cerebral palsy	Growth problems	FTT; overweight due to hypotonia	Constipation	Oral-motor problems	Central nervous system involvement; orthopedic problems; medication–nutrient interactions related to seizure disorder
Down syndrome	Risk for obesity	Related to short stature and hypotonia	Constipation	Poor suck in infancy	Gum disease; increased risk for heart disease, osteoporosis, and Alzheimer's disease
Prader-Willi syndrome	High risk for obesity	FTT in infancy; later obesity related to hypotonia and short stature	N/A	Poor suck in infancy; behavioral feeding/eating problems	Risk for diabetes mellitus
Autism	N/A	N/A	N/A	Limited food selection; sensory feeding/eating problems; behavioral eating/feeding problems	Pica Medication–nutrient interactions
Cystic fibrosis	Underweight	Increased nutrient needs; decreased food intake; decreased absorption of nutrients related to pancreatic insufficiency and chronic pulmonary infection	N/A	N/A	Increase in secondary illnesses: diabetes, liver disease, osteoporosis

(continued)

Table 2.3 *(continued)*

Syndrome/ Disability	Altered Growth, Underweight, Obesity	Altered Energy Needs	Constipation or Diarrhea	Feeding Problems	Other
Spina bifida (myelo- meningocele)	Risk for obesity	Decreased energy needs based on short stature and limited mobility	Constipation	Swallowing problems caused by the Arnold Chiari malformation of the brain	Urinary tract infections
Congenital heart disease	Underweight/ FTT prior to corrective surgeries	Increased needs	N/A	Poor feeding and fatigue prior to surgery	Medications may decrease appetite
Seizure disorder	N/A	N/A	Either may occur due to side effects of certain medications	N/A	Certain medications alter absorption or utilization of nutrients
Attention deficit/ hyperactivity disorder	Possibly underweight due to side effects of certain medications	N/A	N/A	Disruptive mealtimes if untreated	Certain medications can decrease appetite
Cleft lip/palate	N/A	N/A	N/A	Requires use of special nipples if bottle feeding; feedings may be lengthy	

Abbreviations: FTT, failure to thrive; N/A, not applicable.
Source: Data are from references 4 and 5.

Clinical Tips   (*continued from page 26*)

- Clinical judgment is needed when recommending the introduction of solid foods to infants and children who have oral-motor or sensory feeding problems. Recommending ways to adapt how a food is prepared or presented is important. See Chapter 3 for more information on food and feeding adaptations, foods that can cause choking, and developmental feeding topics.
- Baby foods should never be added to infant formula or put in a bottle even if a child is unable to eat these foods by mouth. See Chapter 3 for recommendations concerning feeding infants or children with developmental feeding problems.
- Between 12 and 24 months of age, a child's appetite decreases. The dramatic decrease in food consumption will often alarm parents. It is important to reassure parents that this decrease is normal because the child's rate of growth has slowed considerably. What is needed at this age are small, frequent, and nutrient-dense foods. How the food is presented to a child is important. Using different colors and shapes can encourage a child to eat a variety of nutritious foods. Also emphasize appropriate portion sizes so that the parents do not try to overfeed the child or place too much emphasis on eating portions that are too large. See Chapter 3 for more suggestions on encouraging food intake with toddlers and picky eaters.

Table 2.4
Intake Range for Formula-Fed Premature and Full-Term Infants

Weight Range (lb)	Formula Volume/ Day (fl oz)	No. of Feeding Episodes/Day	Comments
4–5	12–16	8–14	High oral need often confused with hunger until there is a regular sleep/wake cycle
5–6	16–18	6–10	
7–8	18–23	6–10	
8–10	21–26	5–8	Volume per feeding: 3–5 fl oz
10–12	24–28	5–7	Volume per feeding: 3–5 fl oz

Source: Data are from reference 6.

Table 2.5
Typical Feeding Progression and Serving Sizes for Healthy Infants and Toddlers

Age (mo)	Food Group	No. of Servings/Day	Recommended Foods	Typical Serving Size
0–4	Breastmilk and/or formula	8–12	Breastmilk and/or formula	2–4 oz
4–6	Breastmilk and/or formula	4–6	Breastmilk and/or formula	6–8 oz
	Grain	1–2	Infant cereal	1–2 Tbsp
6–8	Breastmilk and/or formula	3–5	Breastmilk and/or formula	6–8 oz
	Grain	2	• Infant cereal • Crackers	• 2–4 Tbsp • 2
	Fruits and vegetables	2 (1 serving juice and 1 serving fruit or vegetable)	• Fruit juice in cup • Fruit or vegetable	• 3 oz • 2–3 Tbsp
8–12	Breastmilk and/or formula, dairy	3–4	• Breast milk and/or formula • Cheese • Yogurt	• 6–8 oz • ½ oz • ½ cup
	Grain	2	• Infant cereal • Bread • Crackers • Pasta	• 2–4 Tbsp • ½ slice • 2 • 3–4 Tbsp
	Fruits and vegetables	3 (2 servings fruit or vegetable and 1 serving juice)	• Fruit or vegetable • Fruit juice in cup	• 3–4 Tbsp • 2–3 oz
	Protein	2	Chicken, beef, pork, beans, or eggs	3–4 Tbsp
12–24	Dairy	3	• Whole milk • Cheese • Yogurt	• 4 fl oz • ½ oz • ½ cup
	Grain	4	• Cereal, pasta, or rice • Bread • Crackers	• ¼ cup • ½ slice • 2
	Fruits and vegetables	4	All fruit or vegetables, cooked or raw	• ¼ cup
	Protein	2	• Chicken, beef, pork • Beans • Eggs	• 1 oz • ¼ cup • 1

Source: Data are from reference 6.

Table 2.6
Feeding Guide for Children

Food	Age 2–3 y	Age 4–6 y	Age 7–12 y	Comments
Milk and dairy				The following may be substituted for ½ cup fluid milk: ½–¾ oz cheese, ½ cup yogurt, 2½ Tbsp nonfat dry milk.
No. of servings	4–5 (16–20 oz total)	3–4 (16–24 oz total)	3–4 (24–32 oz total)	
Portion size	½ cup	½–¾ cup (4–6 oz)	½–1 cup (4–8 oz)	
Meat, fish, poultry, or equivalent				The following may be substituted for 1 oz meat, fish, or poultry: 1 egg, 2 Tbsp peanut butter, 4–5 Tbsp cooked legumes.
No. of servings	2 (2–4 oz total)	2 (2–4 oz total)	3–4 (6–8 oz total)	
Portion size	1–2 oz	1–2 oz	2 oz	
Vegetables and fruits				Include one green leafy or yellow vegetable, such as carrots, spinach, broccoli, winter squash, or greens, for vitamin A.
No. of servings	4–5	4–5	5–6	
Portion size:				
• Cooked vegetables	• 2–3 Tbsp	• ½ cup	• ½ cup	Include one vitamin C–rich fruit, vegetable, or juice: eg, citrus juices, orange, grapefruit, strawberries, melon, tomato, or broccoli.
• Raw vegetables*	• Few pieces	• Few pieces	• Several pieces	
• Raw fruit	• ½–1 small	• 1 small	• 1 medium	
• Canned fruit	• 2–4 Tbsp	• 4–6 Tbsp	• ½ cup	
• Fruit juice	• 3–4 oz	• 4 oz	• 4 oz	
Grain products				The following may be substituted for 1 slice of bread: ½ cup spaghetti, macaroni, noodles, or rice; 5 saltines; ½ English muffin or bagel; 1 tortilla; ½ cup corn grits or posole.
No. of servings	3–4	4–5	5–6	
Portion size:				
• Whole-grain or enriched bread	• ½–1 slice	• 1 slice	• 1 slice	
• Cooked cereal	• ¼–½ cup	• ½ cup	• ½–1 cup	
• Dry cereal	• ½–1 cup	• 1 cup	• 1 cup	

*Do not give to children until they can chew well.
Source: Data are from reference 7.

Dietary Reference Intakes

The dietary reference intakes (DRIs) are a set of nutrient-based reference values that were developed in response to a need for a more precise and customized approach to defining nutrient requirements. The DRIs are a collective term for the following:

- Estimated average requirement (EAR)
- Recommended dietary allowance (RDA)
- Adequate intake (AI)
- Tolerable upper intake level (UL)
- Estimated energy requirement (EER)

The glossary describes each reference set in more detail.

DRIs differ from RDAs in that DRIs aim to improve the long-term health and well-being of a population by making recommendations that will reduce the risk of chronic diseases through improved nutritional intake rather than the prevention of nutritional deficiencies. Health-care providers can obtain more information about DRIs from the Food and Nutrition Board of the Institute of Medicine, National Academy of Sciences Web site (http://www.nap.edu). Table 2.7 includes DRIs for infants and children (9–13).

Calculating Estimated Energy Requirements

To calculate EER for infants and toddlers (birth through 2 years), see Table 2.8 for equations, based on the child's age and weight (13).

Calculating the EER for boys and girls ages 3 to 19 years involves using the age-appropriate equation and inserting the most appropriate physical activity coefficient (PA) into the equation. The PA varies by age, sex, and the degree of activity. Judgments must be made to determine the child's degree of activity. Equations for determining total energy expenditure (TEE) for overweight boys and girls ages 3 to 19 years are also available. TEE can be used by clinicians as an estimate of energy expenditure and to determine energy intakes for children that will result in weight loss or weight maintenance. See Tables 2.9 and 2.10 for EER and TEE equations, and Tables 2.11 and 2.12 for PA coefficients (13). Box 2.1 gives examples of calculating EER and TEE based on current age, weight, height, and PA coefficient.

Recommended Distribution of Macronutrients

It is important to determine the macronutrient distribution (carbohydrate, protein, and fat as a percentage of total energy intake) of an infant or child's diet and then evaluate the distribution using data in Table 2.13 (13). Dietary intakes that

Table 2.7
Dietary Reference Intakes: Recommended Daily Intakes for Individuals*

Nutrient	Infants, 0–6 mo	Infants, 7–12 mo	Children, 1–2 y	Children, 3–6 y	Boys, 9–13 y	Boys, 14–18 y	Girls, 9–13 y	Girls, 14–18 y
Energy (kcal) Active PAL EER[a]	Male: 570 Female: 520 (age 3 mo)	Male: 743 Female: 676 (age 9 mo)	Male: 1,046 Female: 992 (age 24 mo)	Male: 1,742 Female: 1,642 (age 6 y)	2,279 (age 11 y)	3,152 (age 16 y)	2,071 (age 11 y)	2,368 (age 16 y)
Carbohydrate (g)	60	95	130	130	130	130	130	130
Total fiber (g)	ND[b]	ND	19	25	31	48	26	26
Fat (g)	31	30	ND	ND	ND	ND	ND	ND
η-3 polyunsaturated fatty acids (linoleic acid) (g)	4.4	4.6	7	10	12	16	10	11
η-3 polyunsaturated fatty acids (alpha-linoleic acid) (g)	0.5	0.5	0.7	0.9	1.2	1.6	1.0	1.1
Protein (g/kg)	1.5	1.5	1.10	0.95	0.95	0.85	0.95	0.85
Vitamin A (µg)[c]	400	500	300	400	600	900	600	700
Vitamin C (mg)	40	50	15	25	45	75	45	65
Vitamin D (µg)[d,e]	5	5	5	5	5	5	5	5
Vitamin E (mg)[f]	4	5	6	7	11	15	11	15
Vitamin K (µg)	2.0	2.5	30	55	60	75	60	75
Thiamin (mg)	0.2	0.3	0.5	0.6	0.9	1.2	0.9	1.0

(continued)

Table 2.7 (*continued*)

Nutrient	Infants, 0–6 mo	Infants, 7–12 mo	Children, 1–2 y	Children, 3–6 y	Boys, 9–13 y	Boys, 14–18 y	Girls, 9–13 y	Girls, 14–18 y
Riboflavin (mg)	0.3	0.4	0.5	0.6	0.9	1.3	0.9	1.0
Niacin (mg)g	2	4	6	8	12	16	12	14
Vitamin B-6 (mg)	0.1	0.3	0.5	0.6	1.0	1.3	1.0	1.2
Folate (µg)h	65	80	150	200	300	400	300	400
Vitamin B-12 (mg)	0.4	0.5	0.9	1.2	1.8	2.4	1.8	2.4
Pantothenic acid (mg)	1.7	1.8	2	3	4	5	4	5
Biotin (µg)	5	6	8	12	20	25	20	25
Choline (mg)i	125	125	200	250	375	550	375	400
Calcium (mg)	210	270	500	800	1,300	1,300	1,300	1,300
Chromium (µg)	0.2	5.5	11	15	25	35	21	24
Copper (µg)	200	220	340	440	700	890	700	890
Fluoride (mg)	0.01	0.5	0.7	1	2	3	2	2
Iodine (µg)	110	130	90	90	120	150	120	150
Iron (mg)	0.27	11	7	10	8	11	8	15
Magnesium (mg)	30	75	80	130	240	410	240	360
Manganese (mg)	0.003	0.6	1.2	1.5	1.9	2.2	1.6	1.6
Molybdenum (µg)	2	3	17	22	34	43	34	43

Table 2.7 (continued)

Nutrient	Infants, 0–6 mo	Infants, 7–12 mo	Children, 1–2 y	Children, 3–6 y	Boys, 9–13 y	Boys, 14–18 y	Girls, 9–13 y	Girls, 14–18 y
Phosphorus (mg)	100	275	460	500	1,250	1,250	1,250	1,250
Selenium (μg)	15	20	20	30	40	55	40	55
Zinc (mg)	2	3	3	5	8	11	8	9

*This table (using data from the DRI reports, available at: http://www.nap.edu) presents Recommended Dietary Allowances (RDAs) in **bold type** and Adequate Intakes (AI) in ordinary type. RDAs and AIs may both be used as goals for individual intake. RDAs are set to meet the needs of almost all individuals in a group. For healthy breastfed infants, the AI is the mean intake. The AI for other life stages and gender groups is believed to cover needs of all individuals in the group, but lack of data or uncertainty in the data prevent being able to specify with confidence the percentage of individuals covered by this intake.

aEnergy calculated in terms of physical activity level (PAL) and estimated energy requirement (EER). The intake that meets the average energy expenditure of individuals at the reference height, weight, and age.

bND = not determined.

cAs retinol activity equivalents (RAEs). 1 RAE=1 μg retinol, 12 μg β-carotene, 24 μg α-carotene or 24 μg β-cryptoxanthin in foods. To calculate RAEs from retinol equivalents (REs) of provitamin A carotenoids in foods, divide the REs by 2. For preformed vitamin A in foods or supplements and for the provitamin A carotenoids in supplements 1 RE = 1 RAE.

dCholecalciferol. 1 ug cholecalciferol = 40 IU vitamin D.

eIn the absence of adequate exposure to sunlight.

fAs α-tocopherol. α-tocopherol includes RRR α-tocopherol, the only form of α-tocopherol that occurs naturally in foods, and the 2R-stereoisomeric forms of α-tocopherol (RRR-, RSR-, RRS-, and RSS-α-tocopherol) that occur in fortified foods and supplements.

gAs niacin equivalents (NE). 1 mg of niacin = 60 mg of tryptophan; 0–6 months = preformed niacin (not NE).

hAs dietary folate equivalents (DFE). 1 DFE = 1 μg food folate = 0.6 μg of folic acid from fortified food or as a supplement consumed with food = 0.5 μg of a supplement taken on an empty stomach.

iAlthough AIs have been set for choline, there are few data to assess whether a dietary supply of choline is needed at all stages of the life cycle, and it may be that the choline requirement can be met by endogenous synthesis at some of these stages.

Source: Data are from references 9–13.

Table 2.8

Formulas for Calculating Estimated Energy Requirements (EER) (kcal/day) for Infants and Toddlers

Age (months)	Equation
0–3	$(89 \times Wt - 100) + 175$
4–6	$(89 \times Wt - 100) + 56$
7–12	$(89 \times Wt - 100) + 22$
13–35	$(89 \times Wt - 100) + 20$

Abbreviation: Wt, weight (kg).
Source: Data are from reference 13.

Table 2.9

Formulas for Calculating Estimated Energy Requirements (kcal/day) and Total Energy Expenditure (kcal/day) for Boys

Age (y)	Equation
3–8	$EER = 88.5 - 61.9 \times Age\ (y) + PA \times (26.7 \times Wt + 903 \times Ht) + 20$
9–19	$EER = 88.5 - 61.9 \times Age\ (y) + PA \times (26.7 \times Wt + 903 \times Ht) + 25$
3–19, overweight	$TEE = -114 - 50.9 \times Age\ (y) + PA\ (19.5 \times Wt + 1161.4 \times Ht)$

Abbreviations: EER, estimated energy requirement; Ht, height (meters); PA, physical activity coefficient; TEE, total energy expenditure; Wt, weight (kg).
Source: Data are from reference 13.

Table 2.10

Formulas for Calculating Estimated Energy Requirements (kcal/day) and Total Energy Expenditure (kcal/day) for Girls

Age (y)	Equation
3–8	$EER = 135.3 - 30.8 \times Age\ (y) + PA \times (10.0 \times Wt + 934 \times Ht) + 20$
9–19	$EER = 135.3 - 30.8 \times Age\ (y) + PA \times (10.0 \times Wt + 934 \times Ht) + 25$
3–19, overweight	$TEE = 389 - 41.2 \times Age\ (y) + PA \times (15.0 \times Wt + 701 \times Ht)$

Abbreviations: EER, estimated energy requirement; Ht, height (meters); PA, physical activity coefficient; TEE, total energy expenditure; Wt, weight (kg).
Source: Data are from reference 13.

Table 2.11
Physical Activity (PA) Coefficients for Boys
Ages 3 to 19 Years

Activity Level	Coefficient	
	Normal Weight	Overweight
Sedentary	1.0	1.00
Low active	1.13	1.12
Active	1.26	1.24
Very active	1.42	1.45

Source: Data are from reference 13.

Table 2.12
Physical Activity (PA) Coefficients for Girls
Ages 3 to 19 Years

Activity Level	Coefficient	
	Normal Weight	Overweight
Sedentary	1.0	1.00
Low active	1.16	1.18
Active	1.31	1.35
Very active	1.56	1.60

Source: Data are from reference 13.

Table 2.13
Acceptable Macronutrient Distribution Ranges

Age	Range (% of energy)		
	Carbohydrate	Fat	Protein
Full-term infant	35–65	30–55	7–16
1–3 y	45–65	30–40	5–20
4–18 y	45–65	25–35	10–30

Source: Data are from reference 13.

Box 2.1   Examples of Calculating Estimated Energy Intake (EER) and Total Energy Expenditure (TEE)

Example 1:
A girl who is 4 years, 6 months of age, 105.7 cm tall, and weighs 15.3 kg. She plays outside almost every day, rides a tricycle, and watches not more than 2 hours of television per day. (Use formula for girls 3 to 19 years, active PA coefficient.)

EER $= 135.3 - (30.8 \times \text{Age [y]}) + \text{PA} \times (10.0 \times \text{Wt [kg]} + 934 \times \text{Ht [m]}) + 20$
$ = 135.3 - (30.8 \times 4.5) + 1.31 \times (10.0 \times 15.3 + 934 \times 1.057) + 20$
$ = 135.3 - 138.6 + 1.31 \times (153 + 987.2) + 20$
$ = 135.3 - 138.6 + 1493.7 + 20$
$ = 1{,}510 \text{ kcal}$

Example 2:
A boy who is 6 years, 3 months of age, 123.2 cm tall, weighs 39.2 kg, and has a BMI of 25.8 (> 97th percentile). He doesn't like physical activity, avoids recess, has one 15-minute swim lesson per week, and watches 3 to 4 hours television daily. (Use formula for overweight boys, sedentary PA coefficient.)

TEE $= -114 - (50.9 \times \text{Age [y]}) + \text{PA} \times (19.5 \times \text{Wt [kg]} + 1161.4 \times \text{Ht [m]})$
$ = -114 - (50.9 \times 6.25) + 1.00 \times (19.5 \times 39.2 + 1161.4 \times 1.232)$
$ = -114 - 317.5 + 1.00 \times (764.4 + 1430.8)$
$ = -114 - 317.5 + 2195.2$
$ = 1{,}764 \text{ kcal}$

---

are unbalanced can result in short- or long-term complications (for example, a high percentage of fat in an infant formula can result in delayed emptying of stomach contents). For children with special health care needs, altering these recommendations is sometimes needed, and individualized assessment and careful monitoring is important.

Dietary Interventions

Intervention strategies to improve the diets of children with special health care needs include altering energy, macronutrient, micronutrient, fiber, and fluid intake to meet the child's specific needs. Modifying energy intake (either increasing or decreasing) can be accomplished by altering the child's fluid and food intake. Table 2.14 presents methods to increase calories in foods and fluids using food sources (vs commercial products).

Table 2.14
Practical Ways to Increase Energy Intake for Children

Food	kcal	Suggested Uses
Protein		
Peanut butter	94 per Tbsp	On bread, toast, crackers, fruit, vegetables, tortillas, baked goods; in milkshakes, hot cereal
Cheese	120 per oz	On bread, toast, vegetables, pasta, eggs; in salads, dips, sandwiches; mixed into meatloaf, meatballs, soups, potatoes, gravies; as a sauce
Dry milk powder* (instant form)	16 per Tbsp	Added to whole milk, milkshakes, casseroles, spaghetti sauce, meatloaf, gravies, sauces, egg salad, tuna salad, potatoes, macaroni and cheese, puddings, cereals, soups, baked goods
Hummus or bean spread	17 per Tbsp	On bread, crackers, tortillas; as a dip for vegetables; mixed with cheese, potatoes
Milk and dairy products		
Whole milk	20 per fl oz	Add to "instant breakfast," hot chocolate, soups, cooked cereals
Evaporated whole milk	25 per Tbsp	In place of whole milk in desserts, meat dishes, baked goods, milkshakes, soups, and cooked cereals
Ice cream	Approximately 17 per Tbsp (varies with product)	In milkshakes/fruit smoothies; as topping on baked desserts
Cream (heavy)	60 per Tbsp	On cereals, replacement for part of milk in puddings, hot chocolate, milkshakes, baked goods, soups, sauces
Grains		
Wheat germ	25 per Tbsp	In baked goods, casseroles, cereals; toppings for fruit, ice cream; in pancakes
Granola	115 per oz	Topping for yogurt, ice cream, applesauce; as trail mix
Fats, oils, and sweets		
Vegetable oil	110 per Tbsp	In soups, casseroles, vegetables, gravies, cooked cereals, spaghetti sauce
Margarine/ butter	110 per Tbsp	On pancakes, waffles, French toast, bread toast, potatoes, pasta, vegetables; in baked goods, casseroles

(*continued*)

Table 2.14   (*continued*)

Food	kcal	Suggested Uses
Sour cream	25 per Tbsp	On vegetables, potatoes; in casseroles, in dips
Cream cheese	50 per Tbsp	On toast, sandwiches, bagels, baked goods; in dips, scrambled eggs, baked goods
Mayonnaise	100 per Tbsp	On sandwiches, pasta; in salads, deviled eggs, vegetable dips
Chopped nuts[†]	50 per Tbsp	In puddings, salads, casseroles, baked goods; on hot cereals, vegetables, fruits, ice cream
Gravy	26 per Tbsp	On meats, potatoes, pasta, vegetables; in casseroles
Corn syrup	60 per Tbsp	On cereals, fruit; milkshakes, milk
Jams, jellies, syrups	52 per Tbsp	On bread, toast, waffles, pancakes, biscuits, bagels, French toast, ice cream, baked goods
Chocolate syrup, sugar	45 per Tbsp	On ice cream, cereal, waffles, pancakes; in milk drinks, baked goods

*Too much nonfat dry milk should not be added to foods for children younger than 2 years or children with medically complex conditions because it may result in an overload of protein on the kidneys. Check with the physician before recommending this additive.

[†]Do not offer to children younger than 4 years or those who have oral-motor delays because of the risk of choking.

Special Topics Related to Dietary Assessment and Intervention

Estimating Energy Requirements

Standard methods for determining energy requirements for children with special health care needs are used to begin an assessment, but alterations may be necessary due to the child's medical diagnosis. Table 2.15 can be used as a guide to alter estimated energy requirements (14–16).

Medications

Side effects of certain medications can affect appetite, food intake, and eventually growth. Timing of medication and whether the medication should be taken with foods or liquids is important information and can also affect the medication's effectiveness. Some medications can cause digestive problems such as constipation or diarrhea; other medications can deplete nutrients from the body.

Table 2.15

Alternative Methods of Estimating Daily Energy Requirements Based on Health Condition

Medical Diagnosis	Energy Calculation
Down syndrome	For children ages 5 to 11 y: • 14.3 kcal/cm for girls • 16.1 kcal/cm for boys
Spina bifida	For children > 8 y who are minimally active: • To maintain weight: 9–11 kcal/cm or 50% fewer kcal than recommended for a child of the same age without the condition • To promote weight loss: 7 kcal/cm
Prader-Willi syndrome	For all children and adolescents: • 10–11 kcal/cm to maintain growth within a growth channel • 8.5 kcal/cm for slow weight loss and support linear growth
Children with very low energy needs	• Lower: 7–9 kcal/cm • Moderate: 9–11 kcal/cm • High: 12–15 k cal/cm
Failure to thrive	Will depend on etiology or medical condition, but start with EER calculations using ideal body weight for height-age and EER for height-age.*
Cystic fibrosis	Calculate ideal weight based on height, using the pediatric growth chart. Multiply by the child's EER for age. Multiply by a factor of 1.3–1.5 (depending on the severity of the disease) to compensate for increased energy demands.

Abbreviation: EER, estimated energy requirement.

*See Tables 2.8–2.10 for EER formulas. Height-age is defined as age at which current height or length would fall at the 50th percentile on the height-for-age or length-for-age growth chart (see Chapter 1). Ideal body weight for height-age is defined as weight at the 50th percentile for height-age.

Example: 9-month-old old girl with weight of 6.4 kg and length of 66 cm (height-age = 6 months). Ideal body weight for a 6-month-old girl is 7.3 kg.

$$
\begin{aligned}
\text{EER (kcal)} &= (89 \times \text{Wt [kg]} - 100) + 56 \\
&= (89 \times 7.3 - 100) + 56 \\
&= 550 + 56 \\
&= 606
\end{aligned}
$$

Source: Data are from references 14–16.

The long-term use of any medication and the use of multiple medications should be noted in the nutrition assessment, and comments about the consequences documented. Table 2.16 lists some of the most common drug-nutrient interactions of medications used with several chronic conditions of children with special health care needs (3,17).

Food Allergies/Intolerances

Food allergies (also referred to as food hypersensitivities) can be serious and in some cases life-threatening. They are estimated to affect 2% to 8% of the pediatric population and can have serious nutrition implications if major food groups are eliminated from the diet (18). A food allergy is any adverse reaction to an otherwise harmless food or food component that involves the body's immune system. To avoid confusion with other types of adverse reactions to foods, it is important to use the terms "food allergy" or "food hypersensitivity." A food allergy is a result of the body's immune system overreacting to food proteins called allergens.

The most common food allergies are milk and milk products, peanuts, soy, other legumes, tree nuts, eggs, wheat, fish, and shellfish. Children can be allergic to any food. Allergic symptoms can involve the skin, gastrointestinal tract, and the respiratory tract. Treatment is elimination of the food or foods identified by food allergy testing.

The Food Allergy and Anaphylaxis Network (FAAN) (http://www.foodallergy.org) is an excellent resource for both professionals and parents that provides educational materials, recipe books, and other resources. The American Academy of Allergy, Asthma and Immunology (AAAAI) (http://www.aaaai.org) and American College of Allergy, Asthma and Immunology (http://www.acaai.org) are also good resources.

Food intolerances, while not life threatening, can also cause nutrition problems in children due to malabsorption difficulties and gastrointestinal discomfort. The most common food intolerance is lactose intolerance, in which the child lacks the enzyme lactase, which breaks down lactose, the sugar found in milk. Another common intolerance is to gliadin, a constituent of the protein gluten, which is seen in children with celiac disease.

Dietary intervention for both food allergies and food intolerances is the same (see Box 2.2). The food or foods must be eliminated from the diet. Families will need help with the selection of alternative foods to substitute for the foods eliminated to meet energy and nutrient needs. Families will benefit from education in reading food labels to avoid the foods eliminated from the diet. Families will also need support to educate other family members, friends, daycare providers, and schools. Safety plans must be developed for the child with life-threatening food allergies.

Table 2.16
Drug-Nutrient Interactions

Medication	Nutrients Affected	Overall Effect	Prevention of Interaction
Antibiotics	• Minerals • Fats • Protein	Temporary decrease in absorption (resulting from diarrhea, nausea, and/or vomiting); destroys "good" intestinal bacteria flora.	Acidophilus and probiotics may counteract loss of intestinal flora.
Anticonvulsants	• Vitamin D • Vitamin K • Vitamin B-6 • Vitamin B-12 • Folate • Calcium	Decrease nutrient absorption or stores.	Recommend diet high in these nutrients. Vitamin and mineral supplements may be appropriate; seek physician approval.
Cardiac medications (diuretics)	• Potassium • Magnesium • Calcium • Folate	Loss or depletion of nutrient stores; some diuretics can produce these effects; may also cause nausea, diarrhea, and vomiting that lead to reduced food intake.	Recommend foods and fluids high in potassium and magnesium. Suggest strategies to help with decreased appetite.
Corticosteroids (used with asthma, arthritis, gastro-intestinal disease, cardiac disease, cancer, etc)	• Calcium • Phosphorus • Glucose	Long-term use can cause stunting of growth; can deplete calcium and phosphorus that can result in bone loss; can affect glucose levels. May also increase appetite, leading to weight gain.	Monitor weight, laboratory values. Supplement with calcium and vitamin D.
Laxatives	Fat-soluble vitamins	Some are bulking agents and others are laxatives. Some laxatives may deplete fat-soluble vitamins when used long-term.	Encourage a diet high in fiber and fluid to wean child off medication. Check with physician for alternative medication that will not deplete stores.

(continued)

Table 2.16   *(continued)*

Medication	Nutrients Affected	Overall Effect	Prevention of Interaction
Stimulants (used for attention deficit/hyper-activity disorder)		Can decrease appetite, cause weight loss; may affect overall growth.	Have child eat before each medication dosage if possible. Monitor growth and discuss with physician if it is affected.
Sulfonamides (used in spina bifida)	• Vitamin C • Protein • Folate • Iron	Promotes crystalli-zation of large doses of vitamin C in the bladder; inhibits protein synthesis; decreases serum folate and iron.	Avoid supplemen-tation of vitamin C in large doses (> 1000 mg). Increase intake of high-folate foods.
Tranquilizers		Increases appetite; results in excessive weight gain.	Recommend a low-fat diet, if appropriate. Monitor weight.

Source: Data are from references 3 and 17.

Box 2.2   General Guidelines for Nutrition Interventions for Food Allergies and Intolerances

- Confirm that the specific allergy or intolerance has been diagnosed and that the food and food additives have been determined.
- Provide nutrition education and resources to identify the target food.
- Encourage families to share information with child-care and school staff.
- Assure that child-care and school staffs have developed safety plans jointly using the Food Allergy and Anaphylaxis Network guidelines.
- Encourage as much variety in food intake as possible.
- Provide appropriate substitute foods to replace the nutrients missing from the restricted foods.
- When adding new foods, use foods with one ingredient.
- Stress the importance of reading food labels to identify all sources of the restricted food.

Use of Commercial Infant Formulas and Pediatric Nutrition Products

A variety of formulas are now available, varying in composition based on the age of the intended consumer and application, such as an oral supplement or as a total nutrition source from a feeding tube. Typically, infant products are mixed to be 20 kcal per ounce (same energy concentration as breastmilk), whereas toddler and children's products are 30 kcal per ounce. For children older than 10 years of age, review formula requirements on a regular basis to determine if an adult product meets their nutritional needs.

The following factors determine which special formula or complete nutritional supplement is appropriate: age; medical condition; source of macronutrients (protein, fat carbohydrate); renal solute load/osmolality; vitamin, mineral and protein needs; and feeding route (oral or tube).

Typically, a medical specialist or the primary care provider prescribes a special formula (even if it is sold over the counter) to enable possible reimbursement from the child's insurance or other payment systems. Dietetics professionals in the community may be asked to monitor the family's use of the product. Important items to note in follow-up evaluations include gastrointestinal tolerance, weight changes, actual intake as compared with the recommended plan, family's level of satisfaction with the product, and feeding schedule. See Chapter 4 for more information about enteral feedings.

Infant Formula

Breastfeeding for all infants, including those with special needs, is ideal and should be encouraged. Commercial infant formulas are formulated to match breastmilk as much as possible. Modifications can be made to commercial products to alter the nutrients by concentrating the product (ie, using less water) or by adding modular products (eg, protein, carbohydrate, fat). Methods for modification should be recommended and calculated only by pediatric dietetics professionals or specialty physicians and are not included in this chapter. Table 2.17 describes the general categories of infant formulas, energy density, indications for use, and general comments (19).

Pediatric Products for Toddlers and Children

Cow's milk is the beverage of choice for toddlers and children; however, in some cases; special products need to be substituted. These products can be the child's total diet or used as a supplement. See Table 2.17 for more information on pediatric formulas and other supplements, including energy density, indications for use, and general comments.

Table 2.17

Classification of Commercial Formulas: Types and Indications for Use

Category	Indication for Use	kcal/oz (standard dilution)	Comments
Cow's milk infant formula	Infants younger than 1 year. Standard formula when not breastfeeding.	20	Meets FDA infant formula standards
Soy-based infant formula	Infants younger than 1 year who cannot tolerate milk protein or lactose	20	Meets FDA infant formula standard; all are lactose-free; not indicated for the premature infant
Premature infant formula	Premature or LBW infant	22 or 24	Usually short-term use, with transition to regular infant formulas as tolerated; close monitoring after hospital discharge for growth and feeding tolerance recommended. Levels of protein, vitamins, minerals, fat, and carbohydrate vary by product.
Follow-up infant formula	Older infants after solids are introduced or as an alternative to cow's milk	20	Composition varies; some can be used with toddlers; used to "bridge the gap" as solid foods are introduced into the diet.
Hypoallergenic infant formula (casein hydrolysate)	Infants with suspected GI tract damage.	20	Etiology of GI problem determines correct product. Formula has no intact protein but contains amino acids and small peptides. Fat sources vary.
Elemental Infant formula (amino acid-based)	Infants younger than 1 year with suspected cow's milk protein or multiple food-protein allergies.	20	Also used with infants with growth failure due to GERD. Synthetic amino acids are protein source. *(continued)*

Category	Indication for Use	kcal/oz (standard dilution)	Comments
Specialized pediatric (modified protein-based)	Children 1 year or older with chronic GI disorders, food allergies or metabolic diagnoses	20–30	Due to expense generally intended for temporary use if diagnoses will allow (products for metabolic disorders are used for lifetime, with modifications as the child ages). Protein, fat, and carbohydrate sources vary.
Modular products (protein, carbohydrate, fat)	To add calories or nutrients to a standard product	Varies with product	Modulars are used to add either a singular nutrient or combinations (eg, fat and carbohydrate). It is essential to calculate nutrient distribution to assure balance.
Electrolyte and rehydration products	Infants and children; used during acute phases of diarrhea	Varies	Important to instruct parents to follow physician advice and to advance as soon as possible.
Nutrient-dense products	Children 1 year and older unable to maintain adequate oral intake from food. Intact protein, fats, carbohydrates, vitamins and minerals can meet all nutrient needs at specific volume.	30	Many varieties, with flavors, with or without fiber, for oral or non-oral feeding (see also Chapter 4)

Abbreviations: FDA, Food and Drug Administration; GERD, gastroesophageal reflux disease; GI, gastrointestinal; LBW, low birth weight.
Source: Data are from reference 19.

Vitamin and Mineral Supplementation

Some families want to use vitamin and/or mineral supplements even when they are not necessary, eg, when the child has an adequate intake or is receiving a complete nutrition supplement. Parents may ask about the use of a vitamin and/or mineral supplement as an "insurance policy." If the child is eating a variety of

Clinical Tips

- If a special product is used as the child's sole source of nutrition, it is vital to ensure that the child is consuming adequate nutrients (protein, energy, vitamins, minerals, dietary fiber, fluid, etc). The volume needed to meet the child's nutrient needs will vary from product to product. This information must be calculated and the use of computer programs makes this much easier. Calculation and evaluation of the percentage distribution of the major nutrients (carbohydrate, protein, and fat) should meet standards. See Table 2.13.
- To increase the energy density of infant formula, such as making a formula that is 24 kcal/ounce, it is advised to refer to the manufacturer's guidelines. Methods and measuring tools vary with manufacturer.
- When making a large volume of concentrated formula using powder, it may be easier for the family to measure the formula powder in household measuring cups or portions of a cup. Check with the manufacturer for the conversion factors (ie, number of scoops to equal a portion of a measuring cup).
- If an infant or child is consuming a specialized product, be sure to determine how the family is paying for the product. Many of these products are very expensive and families may not be able to pay for the product. State or federal programs can often assist families if needed. See Chapter 6 for more information on ways to obtain reimbursement for specialized products.
- Some children experience gastrointestinal symptoms after a change in nutrition products, even if the nutrient composition seems to be the same. Transition to the new product may involve mixing old and new products or a short-term dilution of the new product. The specialty team or pediatrician needs to be aware of intolerances.
- Formula and complete nutritional supplements should be refrigerated after they are opened and used within 24 hours. Bacterial contamination and subsequent gastrointestinal problems can occur with improperly stored formula, both at home and school.
- The AAP does not recommend the use of low-iron formulas in infant feeding and recommends that all formulas fed to infants be fortified with iron (20). To be labeled "with iron," infant formulas must contain at least 6.7 mg of iron per liter; most standard infant formulas contain approximately 12 mg of iron per liter (20).
- It is important to closely monitor infants and children using specialized formulas or supplements to determine if the child still requires the product. As children grow, their energy and nutrient needs change and the use of the special product should be reassessed. This may be overlooked by others and is the primary responsibility of the dietetics professional.

foods from all of the major food groups, is growing well, and is in overall good health, there is no need for a supplement, even if the child has a chronic disability. However, it may be difficult to determine if the child is growing well if his/her growth pattern is different from established norms, or if the child has periods when he/she does not eat well. The family may benefit from discussing complete multivitamin and mineral supplements or supplements of individual nutrients of special interest, such as calcium or fluoride (refer to Table 2.18) (21).

Generally, the best recommendation is a complete pediatric multivitamin/mineral supplement that meets 100% of the DRIs. A complete pediatric multivitamin/mineral supplement would include zinc, a mineral that is often low in the diet of children with chronic low food intake. The issues of cost, refusal to accept such supplements due to taste, or possible gastrointestinal symptoms should also be discussed with the caregiver. It may be helpful to give the supplement at less than the recommended dose, such as every other day, or only half a tablet.

The DRIs include ULs for many nutrients, based on the potential to cause adverse effects at high levels. This is most often of concern when the high levels of nutrients come from supplements. Cumulative nutrient intake from all sources (food, pediatric formulas, and vitamin/mineral supplements) should be

Table 2.18

Indications for Recommending a Pediatric Vitamin and Mineral Supplement

Condition	Reason
Underweight child with chronic low food intake	Low intake of foods to meet nutrient needs
Child with multiple food allergies	Omission of food groups where nutrients from this food group would typically be obtained
Tube-fed older child with very low energy intake	Low volume due to low energy requirements may limit vitamins and minerals from tube feeding. Crush multivitamin in tube feeding
Child on medications that alter absorption or utilization of certain nutrients	See section on medications
Child with very limited food choices (child with autism, pervasive developmental disorder)	Omission of foods from a food group that provide key nutrients. Often difficult to add a vitamin/mineral supplement because the child will refuse the new item to the diet.

compared with the ULs and appropriate recommendations given to the family to assure safety.

Clinical Tips

- It is helpful to parents to illustrate their child's vitamin or mineral intake by using a computer diet analysis program of a recent intake from a 2- or 3-day food record. Often such an analysis does not show low intakes or the need for supplementation if a commercial product is already being used, but if the product is eliminated from the analysis, the results can be quite compelling.
- Fluoride is recommended for infants and children who do not have access to fluoride in their water supply (ie, families that have well water, have a water supply that is not fluoridated, or use bottled water). Ready-to-feed infant formulas have fluoride added.
- The AAP recommends that exclusively breast-fed infants should receive a supplement to ensure an intake of 200 IU of vitamin D per day. Supplementation should begin within the first 2 months of life (22).
- Calcium, iron, fluoride, and other nutrients that have been reported to be low in diets of healthy children are also likely to be low in children with chronic conditions.
- Families with children with chronic illnesses are more vulnerable to claims from alternative or complementary medicine therapies than other families. If the caregiver is considering the use of a complementary or alternative nutritional therapy for the child, the dietetics professional should document this information in the medical record. Table 2.19 lists information that should be included in the report (21). Because many of these therapies and products are promoted in the mass media and on the Internet, many families of children with special health care needs have difficulty evaluating the usefulness for their child. Health professionals can collaborate with families to identify if the product or therapy is safe to use in children; whether there are any documented reports on effectiveness of the treatment; potential side effects, and the cost, time, and energy required to provide the therapy.

Table 2.19

Nutrition Assessment for Patients Who May Use Complementary or Alternative Nutrition Therapy: Documentation Guidelines

Area of Nutrition Assessment	Reasons for Concern/ Documentation Recommendations
Anthropometric data	Alterations in growth can occur with restricted diets.
Dietary intake	Note any excesses or deficiencies in nutrients and general food categories. Long-term elimination of certain food groups (such as dairy) without compensations can lead to dietary deficiencies (such as calcium and protein).
Food and plant allergies or intolerances	Patients with known plant allergies may exhibit reactions to herbal products from the same category.
Current intake of supplements	It is important to identify the types of supplements the child is currently taking; documentation should include the dosage, duration of use, who recommended the product, and whether the primary physician is aware of use.
Caregiver's plans for implementation	Make note of the proposed treatment the caregivers are considering. Document your responses to the proposed treatment.

Source: Data are from reference 21.

Case Examples

Example 1

Patient

An 8-year-old girl with spastic quadriplegia cerebral palsy.

Problem

Poor growth as a result of low food intake.

Findings

Parents describe feedings as "very difficult" because their daughter fatigues quickly during the meal. The mother estimates that meals consisting of soft, mashed foods typically take about 1 hour. She reports that her daughter has difficulty staying positioned correctly and often falls asleep during the meal. Previous modified barium swallow studies showed that the patient could safely consume thickened liquids without the risk of aspiration. Nutritional supplements and thickeners for fluids had been recommended, but the family did not purchase them because they were so expensive. Based on a 3-day dietary recall, the patient's dietary intake of foods and fluids was well below estimated energy and fluid needs.

Recommendations
- Reassure the mother that she is doing a good job.
- Increase the energy density of the girl's food by adding 1 tablespoon (110 kcal) of margarine, butter, or vegetable oil to her diet. Because there are 3 teaspoons in a tablespoon, one teaspoon can be added to her breakfast, lunch, and dinner meals. Also add grated cheese when possible.
- Initiate referral, with documentation, to the family's insurance company or state agency for Medicaid funding for supplements and thickener.
- Complete a school lunch prescription for modification of the texture and fluids.
- Review history for recent illnesses to determine how the girl's intake decreases with illness and to determine how soon to consider referral for feeding evaluation.

Rationale
Although the patient is likely to need an interdisciplinary feeding evaluation, increasing her energy intake with food and trying to procure the nutritional supplement are the first steps. Supporting the family and identifying funding sources for procuring a complete, nutritional supplement are essential for increasing the patient's energy intake. Identification of supports in school (feeding goals in the Individualized Education Program [IEP], personnel to implement the goals, and modification of school lunch to maximize intake) will also be beneficial.

Example 2

Patient
A 5-year-old boy with autism.

Problem
Self-limited food intake, excessive milk intake.

Findings
Patient will only eat corn chips, bagels, french fries, grapes, and chicken nuggets. He refuses to eat any vegetables, and grapes are the only fruit he will

accept. The boy prefers salty and crunchy foods and foods that are brown or beige in color. He does not like colorful foods, nor does he tolerate any change in his routine. He drinks approximately 40 oz of whole milk per day. A diet analysis indicates he is consuming adequate amounts of protein and calcium (due to milk intake) but his diet is low in iron, zinc, and dietary fiber, and high in fat (chips, french fries, whole milk, chicken nuggets).

Recommendations

- Reassure the mother that she is doing a good job and that food-related issues are often seen in children with autism.
- The goal is to improve the nutrient quality of the diet by expanding the variety of foods consumed.
- Have the family offer the patient some of the preferred brown/beige salty and crunchy foods, then begin to slowly add other items. (A mix of corn chips and peanuts was introduced and accepted. Gradually, fortified dry cereals, raisins, dried apricots, and granola were added. Also, turkey served with the patient's favorite gravy was introduced and accepted.)
- A chewable multivitamin/mineral supplement that is brown/beige in color may be accepted.
- Recommend the use of low-fat foods, especially low-fat milk. This may need to be a gradual process of mixing whole milk with low-fat milk at different ratios.
- With permission from the parents, make a referral to a feeding specialist or the child's school team to provide sensory or behavioral therapy to assist him in accepting a greater variety of foods.
- Provide suggested goals for the family to incorporate in the child's IEP, eg, increased tolerance or acceptance of more food variety, consistent approach to snack environment.

Rationale

A self-restricted diet is often observed with the diagnosis of autism, and improving the quality of the child's diet requires a team approach. His sensory-related eating problems and rigid routine are the cause of his limited food intake, and the behavioral aspects of his condition are compounding the problem. Maintenance of the patient's mealtime routines is important while the dietary changes are being made.

Example 3

Patient

A 7-year-old boy with midlevel spina bifida.

Problem
Child is overweight.

Findings
The boy has limited mobility and uses crutches and leg braces. His IEP includes a generalized education setting with special education services. He is short for his age, and his body mass index (BMI) is above the 90th percentile. He has a great appetite, but refuses to eat whole-wheat bread, raw vegetables, and fruits that were previously recommended to increase the dietary fiber content of his diet to help prevent chronic constipation. He drinks 3 to 4 cups of cranberry juice per day and loves hot dogs, potato chips, pasta, and sweets. His favorite leisure-time activities include watching television and playing computer games.

Recommendations
- Recommend the use of low-fat foods for meals and snacks and provide the family with specific examples and choices.
- Recommend other fluid options to reduce the excessive juice consumption while maintaining overall fluid intake, which is important for bowel and bladder function. Suggest the use of water and diet cranberry juice instead.
- Provide education concerning correct portion sizes. Discuss strategies to discourage large portions (pre-plate meals, use smaller plates and bowls, etc) and urge that the whole family be involved.
- Encourage increased activity, with his participation in community recreation options or Special Olympics, as well as family activities such as swimming or rowing.
- Confirm that the family is aware of the spina bifida support group because this group may act as a resource for community activities.

Rationale
This patient's overweight is the result, in part, of his body composition (decreased muscle in the lower limbs) and decreased activity due to the necessity of using crutches to ambulate. As a result, he requires less energy than other children his age. Nutrition education for the child and family should focus on the consumption of low-fat, low-calorie food choices. Encouraging leisure-time activities that require movement and activity in inclusive settings will be a long-term goal. Educate the parents that a focus should be controlling energy intake and portion control, rather than increasing dietary fiber, because an increase in dietary fiber is not as effective as medication in treating the type of constipation seen in spina bifida.

Example 4

Patient

An infant with a congenital heart condition who has just undergone surgery and is receiving cardiac medications.

Problem

Infant is a poor feeder who falls asleep after a few ounces; weight gain is slow. The mother requests assistance to help her daughter gain weight and eat better.

Findings

The mother is correctly making and offering 24 kcal/oz formula. She has been urged by concerned relatives to add cereal to her infant's diet even though the specialty team at the cardiac clinic discouraged this practice.

Recommendations

- Reassure the mother that following recommendations of the specialty team is the right thing to do. Offer to contact the physician on the specialty team to let him know of the mother's concerns and discuss other options that the team would recommend.
- Nutritional quality of infant's diet can be improved with modular products to increase energy density; however, this infant should be referred back to the cardiac specialist.

Rationale

The infant's specialty care team should recommend any formula changes, because the infant's fatigue may be related to the cardiac condition itself and/or required medications. The role of the community team is to support the family in following through with the specialty team's recommendations.

Example 5

Patient

A 15-month-old boy with multiple food allergies to wheat, dairy, egg, peanuts, and beef.

Problem

Poor growth and limited food choices.

Findings

Food record reveals that the child's diet is low in energy, protein, iron, calcium, and other nutrients. His mother reports that her son will only eat rice cakes, rice puffs, chicken, and apples. He will only drink juices and rice milk. When offered new foods he usually will take just one bite and spit it out. He is often irritable and wakes frequently at night.

Recommendations

- Recommend trying an elemental formula designed for toddlers to increase energy and nutrients in the diet. This should be offered as the only beverage to improve the child's nutritional status. Suggest strategies for helping the mother deal with the child's temper tantrums for juice.
- Increase energy by fortifying food with nondairy margarine or vegetable oil.
- Make sure the family is aware of the Food Allergy and Anaphylaxis Network (http://www.foodallergy.org) as a valuable support.
- Create a list of safe snack foods and review label reading.
- Obtain permission from the mother to review the case with child's allergist to be sure that there are no other food allergies. Determine the allergist's plan for introducing new foods and your involvement in this plan.

Rationale

This child may have other food allergies; therefore, it is important to discuss this with the child's allergist. The child needs to consume an elemental formula to improve his nutritional status. It is important to review label reading with the family because they may be unknowingly giving foods with wheat, dairy, eggs, peanuts, or beef.

References

1. Campbell MK, Kelsey KS. The PEACH survey: a nutrition screening tool for use in early intervention programs. *J Am Diet Assoc.* 1994;94:1156–1158.
2. Baer MT, Harris AB. Pediatric nutrition assessment: identifying children at risk. *J Am Diet Assoc.* 1997;97(10 Suppl 2):S107-S115.
3. Nardella M, Campo L, Ogata B, eds. *Nutrition Interventions for Children With Special Health Care Needs.* Olympia, Wash: Washington State Department of Health; 2002.
4. Position of the American Dietetic Association: providing nutrition services for infants, children and adults with developmental disabilities and special health care needs. *J Am Diet Assoc.* 2004;104:97–107.
5. Baer MT, Farnan S, Mauer AM. Children with special health care needs. In: Sharbaugh C, ed. *Call to Action.* Washington, DC: National Center for Education in Maternal and Child Health; 1990:192–207.
6. Department of Nutrition and Food Service. *Pediatric Nutrition Handbook.* 3rd ed. Boston: Mass: Boston Children's Hospital; 1993.

7. Feeding the child. In: Kleinman RE, ed. Committee on Nutrition, American Academy of Pediatrics. *Pediatric Nutrition Handbook.* 5th ed. Elk Grove Village, Ill: American Academy of Pediatrics; 2004:119–136.

8. American Academy of Pediatrics, Committee on Nutrition. The use and misuse of fruit juice in pediatrics. *Pediatrics.* 2001;107:1210–1213.

9. Institute of Medicine. *Dietary Reference Intakes for Calcium, Phosphorus, Magnesium, Vitamin D, and Fluoride.* Washington, DC: National Academy Press; 1997.

10. Institute of Medicine. *Dietary Reference Intakes for Thiamine, Riboflavin, Niacin, Vitamin B6, Folate, Vitamin B12, Pantothenic Acid, Biotin, and Choline.* Washington, DC: National Academy Press; 1998.

11. Institute of Medicine. *Dietary Reference Intakes for Vitamin A, Vitamin K, Arsenic, Boron, Chromium, Copper, Iodine, Iron, Manganese, Molybdenum, Nickel, Silicon, Vanadium and Zinc.* Washington, DC: National Academy Press; 2001.

12. Institute of Medicine. *Dietary Reference Intakes for Vitamin C, Vitamin E, Selenium, and Carotenoids.* Washington, DC: National Academy Press; 2000.

13. Institute of Medicine. *Dietary Reference Intakes for Energy, Carbohydrate, Fat, Fatty Acids, Cholesterol, Protein, Fiber, and Amino Acids.* Washington, DC: National Academy Press; 2002.

14. Story M, Holt K, Sofka D, eds. *Bright Futures in Practice: Nutrition.* Arlington, Va: National Center for Education in Maternal and Child Health; 2000.

15. Sandrock M. Feeding the child with very low energy needs. *Nutrition Focus.* 1997;12(1):1–8.

16. Peterson K, Washington JS, Rathbun J. Team management of failure to thrive, *J Am Diet Assoc.* 1984:810–815.

17. Nutrition management of seizure disorders. In: Nevin-Folino N, ed. *Pediatric Manual of Clinical Dietetics.* 2nd ed. Chicago, Ill: American Dietetic Association; 2003:423–450.

18. Food hypersensitivity. In: Kleinman RE, ed. *Pediatric Nutrition Handbook.* 5th ed. Elk Grove Village, Ill: American Academy of Pediatrics; 2004:593–607.

19. Hattner JT. Pediatric formula update 2004. *Nutrition Focus.* 2004;19(1):1–7.

20. American Academy of Pediatrics, Committee on Nutrition. Iron-fortified infant formulas. *Pediatrics.* 1999;104:119–123.

21. Holland M. Communicating with families concerning the use of complementary or alternative nutritional therapies. *Building Block for Life.* 2000; 24:6–11.

22. Vitamins. In: Kleinman RE, ed. *Pediatric Nutrition Handbook.* 5th ed. Elk Grove Village, Ill: American Academy of Pediatrics; 2004:339–365.

Chapter 3

Feeding and Eating

Maria T. Nardella, MA, RD, and Aaron Owens-Kuehner, MS, RD

Developmental Stages: What to Expect

Typical Feeding Skill Development

Development of feeding behavior depends on the maturation of the central nervous system, which controls the acquisition of fine, gross, and oral-motor skills. Each of these skills influences the child's ability to consume food. The general terms used to describe the oral-motor feeding process include sucking, swallowing, chewing, gagging, tongue lateralization, and biting (1).

Healthy neonates use a variety of cries and vocalizations to express their needs to caregivers. Parents develop positive interactions with their infants when they are sensitive to, and respond appropriately to, feeding-related behavioral cues. Parents must learn to recognize hunger and satiation in infants and be willing to accept their infant's expressive cues. A lactation specialist or neonatal nurse can be a valuable resource in helping parents learn to read their newborn's cues.

Oral-Motor and Developmental Stages of Readiness in Eating

Understanding normal oral-motor development is essential for assessing children who demonstrate feeding problems. The typically developing infant is born ready to suck. By 18 months of age, the same infant has developed all of the oral movements needed for feeding, except refined rotary jaw movement. The growth and development for all oral skills is believed to continue until approximately the age of 3 years (1,2). After this point, the typically developed child should have all the basic oral skills that will be needed as an adult. Typical development of feeding skills proceeds in an orderly and predictable sequence. Foods should be introduced to match the developmental skill level of the child. See Table 3.1 for the typical development of feeding skills (1,2).

Table 3.1

Typical Development of Feeding Skills

Age (mo)	Oral-Motor Skills	Self-Feeding Skills	Food Transitions
Birth	• Able to suck from the breast or bottle		
1–2	• Suckling strong • Tongue moves forward and back		
2–4	• Corners of lips become active in sucking • Head control initiated • Tongue protrudes, mouth opens in anticipation	• Begins reaching for objects	
4–6	• Voluntary sucking begins • More mature trunk control • Munching pattern emerges • Tongue voluntarily projects outward • Purses and smacks lips	• Recognizes breast/ bottle • Puts hand on bottle • Mouths objects	• May begin strained foods by spoon
6–8	• Lips close around spoon • Vertical chewing begins • Tongue lateralization emerges • Munching continues	• Able to sit alone • Begins to hold bottle • Plays with spoon • Brings food to mouth • Begins to sip from a cup • Voluntary release and resecure of hand-held objects	• Progression of solid food continues • Add large, soft finger foods • Begin to offer juice/formula from a cup
8–10	• Voluntary bite emerges • Tongue begins to move independently from jaw • Transfers food from center to sides of mouth • Lip closure achieved	• Can finger feed with palmar grasp • Can hold own bottle • Sips from a cup	• Decrease use of strained foods • Add finely chopped or mashed table foods • Formula/juice in cup

(*continued*)

Age (mo)	Oral-Motor Skills	Self-Feeding Skills	Food Transitions
10–12	• Rotary chewing begins • Closes lips when swallowing • Licks food from lower lip • Increased tongue and lip control	• Begins to hold cup • Finger-feed with pincer grasp • Bites food • Begins self-feeding with spoon	• Add small finger foods • Add chopped table foods
12–15	• Takes 4–5 continuous swallows of liquid • Improved rotary chewing	• Drinking from a cup at all meals • Practice with spoon improves	• Progression of textured table foods continues • Begin to wean from bottle; more cup drinking
18–36	• Development of all oral movements needed for feeding, except refined rotary jaw movement • Skills believed to continue to develop until this point	• More practice and maturity with skills	• Regular table foods • Weaned from bottle; liquids in cup • Take caution with foods that may cause choking *
> 36	• All basic oral skills needed as an adult are present		

*For example, raw vegetables, nuts, hot dogs, popcorn.
Source: Data are from references 1 and 2.

Matching Appropriate Feeding Advancement with Developmental Milestones

Infants and children with developmental delays may also be delayed in their development of eating skills. Oral-motor activity involves body positioning, fine and gross motor skills, social interactions, and cognitive level, any of which may be negatively affected by a child's overriding medical condition. Anticipatory guidance for parents regarding developmental changes is important in advancing appropriate feeding skills and behaviors.

Clinical Tip

The ability of the child, not the chronological age, should dictate the oral feeding stage. However, infant foods are not nutritionally dense enough for the older child, even if the texture is appropriate. Table foods that have been blended may be more appropriate.

Feeding Behaviors: An Overview

Common Feeding and Eating Behaviors: Infants and Nonverbal Children

In a typical feeding situation, the infant is in control of his or her food and fluid intake by communicating hunger and satiety cues to the caregiver. As infants mature, they respond to their feeder's reaction to the cues they provide (1). This response may be positive or negative, causing either a decrease or increase of a certain feeding behavior, depending on the feeder's reaction to the infant. See Table 3.2 for further guidance on feeding interactions (3).

Appetite and Eating Behavior Distortions

Infants and children with developmental delays will give cues to caregivers about hunger and fullness, but they may be subtle and nonverbal. It can be challenging for a parent to recognize these expressive cues. If a positive response to

Table 3.2
Infant-Caregiver Feeding Interactions

Infant Activity	Appropriate Feeder Response
Cries or whimpers	Initiate feeding
Opens mouth in anticipation	Continue feeding
Smacks lips after each spoonful	Continue feeding
Turns head away from spoon	Stop feeding
Averts eyes	Stop feeding
Pushes spoon away	Stop feeding

Source: Data are from reference 3.

a hunger cue is not received, infants may stop attempting to give any signals of hunger and underfeeding may result. Conversely, caregivers may give food to satisfy all types of infant discomforts. Infants, in turn, may not learn to discriminate hunger from other discomforts and rely on eating to satisfy a wide variety of needs (1). Some infants and children may have a distorted sense of hunger and satiety and may develop unusual feeding behaviors as a result of their medical condition.

Clinical Tips

An infant with few hunger cues may not wake up during the night to feed. Parents may need to wake the infant on a schedule, at least until the hunger sensation "kicks in." Anecdotally, some children who are reluctant eaters are reported to have been "good sleepers" as infants and to have slept through the night at an early age. Satiety cues for infants and nonverbal children include the following (1,3):

- Draws head away from nipple
- Fusses or cries during feeding
- Averts gaze away from feeding
- Blocks mouth with hands
- Changes posture
- Keeps mouth tightly closed
- Shakes head as if to say "no"
- Hands become more active
- Sputters with tongue and lips
- Falls asleep

Encouraging parents to be their child's best advocate should begin early. Help new parents become confident in their ability to describe their baby's feeding abilities and recognize changes that might improve treatment plans, especially when many health care providers are involved.

Common Feeding and Eating Behaviors: Older Infants and Children

When a caregiver is extremely anxious about a child's food intake, it is common for children to use negative food-related behaviors, much like those listed in Table 3.3, as a way to manipulate and gain control. This can be a significant problem in children who have conditions that result in oral-feeding problems and/or altered nutritional needs.

Table 3.3
Positive and Negative Feeding Behaviors

Positive Feeding Behaviors	Negative Feeding Behaviors
• Acceptance of a wide variety of foods and textures • Self-feeding at appropriate developmental level • Remaining seated during mealtime • Eating at a moderate pace • Eating and drinking quietly • Using eating utensils appropriately • Chewing and swallowing with the mouth closed	• Crying when food is offered • Refusal to accept food • Throwing food • Gagging and vomiting in response to food offered • Inability or unwillingness to sit still during mealtime

Clinical Tip

Behavioral problems are more common in children with special health care needs and chronic illnesses such as cystic fibrosis and diabetes because the parent and child may be struggling with control issues at mealtimes. The first step in the intervention is to separate food-related behavior and parent-child interactions.

Sometimes parents misinterpret a child's oral-motor problem as "bad" behavior or lack of appetite, rather than recognizing that the child may not be developmentally ready for a specific food.

Feeding Problems and Associated Conditions

Feeding problems are defined as the inability or refusal to eat certain foods because of neuromotor dysfunction, obstructive lesions, or psychological factors. Problems generally are classified as oral-motor, positioning, and behavioral (1,2).

Adjustments for Children with Special Health Care Needs

Feeding and eating problems are more common in children with special health care needs than in the general pediatric population (2). Assessment should be as comprehensive as possible to determine the causes and extent of the problem, so that effective interventions can be implemented. Refer to Table 3.4 for assis-

Table 3.4
Identification and Consequences of Feeding Problems

Presenting Concerns	Possible Causes	Consequences
• Hypersensitivity to touch or temperature in and around the mouth • Poor suck • Drooling • Poor lip closure around nipple, spoon, or rim of cup • Retention of primitive reflexes (rooting reflex) • Abnormal reflexes (tonic bite reflex) • Hypersensitive gag reflex • Anatomical abnormalities that interfere with feeding (cleft lip/palate) • Severe dental caries • Lack of variety in diet • Refuses to eat • Chokes or gags on food • Inadequate intake • Inadequate weight gain, with or without illness • Not weaning despite reasonable effort • Behavioral problems such as irritability	• Problems recognizing hunger and satiety • Developmental problems such as mental retardation • Medical basis for feeding-problem • Swallowing or gastrointestinal dysfunction • Gastroesophageal reflux disease • Positioning problem • Dental problem causing oral pain • Anatomical problem of the mouth, gums, palate, or jaw • Fatigue, depression, or other psychological problem • Behavioral problem such as distractibility • Food insecurity • Lack of parent knowledge/resources	• Slow growth • Inadequate weight gain • Dental caries • Anemia and other vitamin and mineral deficiencies • Psychosocial and interaction problems • Inability to progress to textured foods • Refusal to consume specific foods, types of foods, or food groups • Appetite distortions • Dehydration and/or constipation • Behavioral problems such as irritability

Source: Data are from references 1, 2, and 4.

tance in identifying feeding problems and their possible causes and consequences (1,2,4).

Common Oral-Motor Feeding Problems
Frequently, children with feeding problems exhibit delayed oral-motor development involving the abnormal persistence of primitive movements such as the rooting reflex, the phasic bite reflex, suckling, and inadequate jaw grading. Delayed feeding development may also be related to inadequate structure or

strength of the oral mechanism, or abnormal muscle tone (1). For example, children with Down syndrome demonstrate poor lip closure associated with hypotonia. Infants with cleft lip and palate frequently lack the structural requirement for efficient sucking. Some children with feeding problems have abnormal oral-motor patterns rarely seen and need to be referred to a therapist. See Table 3.5 for common oral-motor feeding problems (1) and Table 3.6 for common diagnoses associated with feeding problems (2,4).

Prematurity: Consequences on Feeding Skill Development and Behavior

Healthy but premature and low-birth-weight infants have a range of feeding problems that are less likely to be seen in full-term infants (2,5). Accurate assessment of corrected age is useful in establishing nutritional and feeding goals and anticipating potential difficulties.

Extended hospitalization may alter the infant-caregiver feeding experience for premature infants. The infants may have multiple feeders, and parents may have limited feeding opportunities. Adequate growth and feeding are often the final criteria for hospital discharge, and parents may be anxious about weight gain.

Table 3.5
Common Oral-Motor Feeding Problems

Feeding Problem	Description
Tonic bite reflex	Strong, involuntary jaw closure when teeth and gums are stimulated
Tongue thrust	Forceful and repetitive protrusion of an often bunched or thickened tongue in response to oral stimulation
Jaw thrust	Forceful opening of the jaw to the maximal extent during eating, drinking, attempts to speak, or general excitement
Tongue retraction	Pulling back the tongue within the oral cavity on the presentation of food, spoon, or cup
Lip retraction	Pulling back the lips in a very tight smile-like pattern at the approach of a stimulus toward the face
Nasal regurgitation	Movement of oral contents up into the nose and lower sinus during swallowing
Sensory defensiveness	A strong adverse reaction to touch, light, or sound

Source: Data are from reference 1.

Table 3.6
Common Diagnoses and Conditions Associated With Feeding Problems

Diagnosis	Behavior	Possible Nutritional Consequences
Premature or very-low-birth weight infant	Subtle and delayed hunger cues from infants, difficult for parent to recognize	Sleepy or irritable infant with slow weight gain
Autism	Rigid food acceptance; picky eating	Nutrient deficiency
Infants of mothers with substance abuse	Non-nutritive need to suck; overfeeding	Excessive weight gain
Down syndrome	Poor suck/feeding in infancy Overfeeding/overeating in older children	Failure to thrive Overweight or obesity
Fetal alcohol syndrome	Distorted hunger perception; undereating	Underweight
Spina bifida	Overfeeding/overeating with limited activity	Overweight or obesity
Neurological impairments	Limited hunger cues; underfeeding	Failure to thrive
Prader-Willi syndrome, older child	Distorted sense of hunger/ satiety; overeating	Excessive weight gain or obesity

Source: Data are from references 2 and 4.

After discharge, some infants may experience setbacks in feeding and growth. Provision of information about a premature infant's feeding skills, nutrition needs, and growth expectations may facilitate the transition home and relieve parents' anxiety. The nutrient requirements of premature infants are generally higher than those of full-term infants because of limited body stores, metabolic and physiological immaturity, and increased growth rates (5). Nipple feeding may increase energy expenditure in some infants. Many premature babies have had negative oral experiences or limited mouth play, making them extra sensitive to changes in their mouths (2). Moving from strained foods to textured or lumpy foods may be very upsetting. Refer to Table 3.7 (2,5) and Box 3.1 (1,6–9) for more information about this subject.

Table 3.7

Developmental Maturity and Nutritional Implications for Premature Infants

Developmental Factor	Nutritional Implications
Immature suck-swallow-breathe coordination emerges between 33 and 36 weeks gestational age	• Impaired nippling ability • Increased risk of aspiration • Decreased feeding efficiency • Fatigue
Diminished or absent gag and cough reflex	• Increased risk of aspiration
Decreased muscle tone	• Inability to maintain optimal feeding position
Neurological and behavioral immaturity	• Subtle cues of hunger, satiety, and distress • More time spent sleeping • Less time alert for feedings • Disorganized feeding skills
Immature peristaltic and gastrointestinal motility patterns	• Delayed gastric emptying • Increased transit time • Constipation
Decreased or absent sucking pads	• Decreased sucking strength and stamina
Reduced gastric volume	• Volume limitations
Lower levels of lactase in infants born at less than 34 weeks' gestation	• Potential for lactose malabsorption
Lower lipase and bile acid levels	• Potential for long-chain fat malabsorption
Alterations in renal and cardiac function	• Fluid and electrolyte imbalance • Alteration in protein tolerance

Source: Data are from references 2 and 5.

Gastroesophageal Reflux Disease

Gastroesophageal reflux disease (GERD) is a condition in which the contents of the stomach seep back into the esophagus and/or throat (2). It may be described as "spitting up, vomiting, or retching." It occurs when the sphincter between the stomach and esophagus is not mature yet or does not function properly. The seepage results in a burning sensation in the esophagus and discomfort similar to heartburn. If the stomach contents seep all the way to the throat, they can enter the child's airway and cause aspiration. Presenting symptoms can vary from occasional regurgitation to persistent or projectile vomiting.

Box 3.1   Ways to Promote Feeding for Premature Infants

- Offer breast milk, fortified breast milk, or nutritionally appropriate formula.
- Offer small, frequent feedings.
- Create a calm feeding environment (quiet room, low light).
- Help prepare infant for feeding (swaddling, thumb sucking).
- Establish a position to improve suck (chin tucked slightly, head supported, one or both arms forward, straight trunk, bent hips).
- Stabilize cheek and lips (gently draw cheeks forward).
- Support jaw.
- Try special feeding equipment (soft nipple, angled-neck bottle).

Source: Data are from references 1, 6–9.

The discomfort resulting from GERD may come to be associated with feedings. Some children may refuse to eat, stop eating after only a small amount of food, cry, become irritable, or use other behavior to communicate their distress. Although healthy infants commonly outgrow GERD, some children with neurological impairments have this problem diagnosed after infancy when it may continue and be more severe (1). Surgery for GERD is infrequent for infants, but is more likely in older children with neurologic disabilities.

If an obvious reason for food refusal cannot be determined, GERD is a likely explanation. If GERD has been previously diagnosed, a medication schedule or dosage change may be needed. Parents often think that GERD has resolved, when in reality the condition may vary over time from dormancy to active irritation in some children.

It should be noted that some studies have disputed the effectiveness of non-surgical treatments such as positioning and thickened feedings for treatment of reflux in healthy, full-term infants (10). However, nonsurgical interventions may be worth trying for infants and children with other medical complications. See Table 3.8 for information on assessment of GERD patients (1,11).

Clinical Tip

Secondhand tobacco smoke can alter lower esophageal sphincter pressure and promote reflux. This is one more reason to eliminate smoke from a child's environment.

Table 3.8

Gastroesophageal Reflux Disease: Assessment and Intervention

Assessment	Possible Interventions
• History of frequent spitting up, choking, coughing, or difficulties with breathing during and after meals • Food refusal • History of repeated upper respiratory infections and pneumonia • Positive finding on upper gastro-intestinal studies, pH probe, or in response to medication	• Upright positioning; elevated sleeping position • Change mealtime volume and timing (smaller, more frequent feedings) • Thicken liquids and foods • Prescription medication • Surgical correction such as fundoplication

Source: Data are from references 1 and 11.

Swallowing Problems

Effective eating requires an efficient and safe swallow. Because swallowing dysfunction can lead to aspiration, difficulties in swallowing function not only influence children's food intake and thus their nutrition, but also may impact their overall health. Therefore, an assessment of the swallowing function should occur during a screening of the motor skills necessary for eating. See Table 3.9 for information on the assessment of swallowing dysfunction (1,4,12,13).

Clinical Tip

The modified barium swallow test is used to document dysphagia (4). Results are most helpful if different types of food textures are used and the staff administering the test has pediatric experience. If results indicate that major changes in feeding are required, providing a copy of the videotape to the feeding therapists and the family may assist in implementing the recommendations.

Some children have an easier time organizing a safe swallow with thicker liquids (refer to Table 3.10 [14]). Some children's swallowing abilities change over time, particularly with the correction of failure to thrive and improved head positioning. Repeat swallowing studies should be considered, especially if parents think that there have been changes.

It is important to tell families in advance that swallowing studies may show that it is medically unsafe to continue oral feeding. Allow the family time to prepare if nonoral feeding may be needed.

Table 3.9
Swallowing Dysfunction: Assessment and Intervention

Assessment	Interventions
• History of frequent spitting up, choking, coughing, or difficulties with breathing during and after meals • History of repeated upper respiratory infections and pneumonia • Noisy or wet sounding upper airway sounds • Drooling or pooling of saliva • More than one swallow needed to clear a bolus • Modified barium swallow study (variation of upper gastrointestinal study)	• If risk of aspiration is documented, refer for nonoral feeding interventions. It is unsafe to make oral feeding recommendations if the risk of aspiration is identified. • Refer to a qualified therapist (speech, occupational therapist) for specific techniques. • Refer to a specialty feeding team. • Evaluate the feeding pace and positions that enhance safe swallowing.

Source: Data are from references 1, 4, 12, and 13.

Clinical Tip

Some thickeners bind part of the fluid, decreasing its bioavailability. It is essential for water intake to be assessed in children with special needs who have problems with drinking fluids (14). Poor hydration can lead to constipation and concentration of urine.

Medications: Additional Effects on Feeding and Eating

Many children with special needs take medications, which may present more challenges to feeding, eating, and nutritional status (2,15). Some medications can

- Depress or increase appetite
- Distort taste
- Reduce alertness
- Alter the swallow reflex
- Cause nausea
- Produce dryness of the oral mucosa
- Irritate the gastrointestinal tract
- Result in malabsorption of vitamins and nutrients
- Cause constipation

Refer to Chapter 2 for further issues relating to nutrition and medication.

Table 3.10
Thickening Products

Food/Product	kcal	Used With Liquids	Used With Foods
Widely available foods			
Pureed or blenderized fruits and/or vegetables	5–11/Tbsp	X	
Infant cereal	15/Tbsp	X	X
Yogurt	8–15/Tbsp	X	
Soft tofu	10/Tbsp	X	
Potato flakes	11/Tbsp		X
Wheat germ	27/Tbsp		X
Bread crumbs	22/Tbsp		X
*Commercial products**			
Thick-It/Thick-It 2	16/Tbsp	X	X
Simply Thick—nectar consistency	0 per 8 oz of fluid	X	X
Simply Thick—honey consistency	5 per 8 oz of fluid	X	X
NutraThik	20/Tbsp	X	X
Thick & Easy	15/Tbsp	X	X

*Thick-It, Alberto-Culver, USA, Melrose Park, IL 60160; Simply Thick, Simply Thick, LLC, St. Louis, MO 63105; NutraThik and Thick & Easy, Hormel Foods Corp, Austin, MN 55912.
Source: Data are from reference 14.

Assessment and Interventions

The interventions described in this chapter are related to promoting feeding skill development, feeding behavior, the feeding environment, and the feeder's sensitivity to the child's eating cues. Intervention for each oral-motor problem differs, depending on the nature of the problem and the developmental level of the child. The use of an interdisciplinary team, with the caregiver as a member of the team, facilitates intervention. Refer to Table 3.11 for assessment of feeding problems and Table 3.12 for the behavioral models of feeding stimulation.

Table 3.11

Assessment of Feeding Problems

Observation	Interview
• Positioning, length of time of the feeding • Portion size offered • Amount of food consumed • Amount of liquid served and consumed • Appetite and signs of hunger or fullness • Rate of eating and drinking • How food is refused • Feeding utensils used • Interaction between the child and feeder	• Types of food eaten (texture, consistency) • Number of feedings per day • Food allergies/intolerances • Use of supplements, herbal preparations, and alternative therapies • Sources of food and formulas, such as WIC, school, or other programs • Medications taken • Sources of family stress or concern, such as child care

Abbreviation: WIC, Special Supplemental Nutrition Program for Women, Infants, and Children.

Table 3.12

Behavioral Models of Feeding Skills

General Objective	Example
Identify the developmental level for a specific skill in one feeding component, such as self-feeding, oral-motor skills, or meal pattern.	The child's oral-motor skills are at 8 months with resistance to most textured foods.
Identify the signs of readiness for the next developmental step in that one area.	The child will look at and open mouth for a spoon of food.
Reinforce the signs of readiness for the new skill consistently by praise or an age-appropriate reward.	Feeder adds tiny soft lumps to accepted foods, or thickens strained foods (with dried baby cereal, instant potatoes, etc) and praises the child after a taste.
Practice and repeat the new skill until it is achieved, then discontinue the reward.	Feeder offers new texture slowly, starting with well-liked foods or a new food with familiar taste and texture. Feeder will grind familiar foods to create a new texture. Use foods that stick together (eg, oatmeal, blended casseroles).

Clinical Tips

One of the most valuable techniques for assessing a child with feeding problems is to observe the caregiver feeding the child in the home environment, or at least in an environment familiar to the child.

Often children with special health care needs have more feeding and eating problems in public than when they are at home. However, never being able to eat in public can lead to isolation rather than needed social acceptance and support.

Some children eat better for one family member than another. If possible, observe the family members as they feed the child to determine if cues or interactions are creating a behavior problem. If the less successful feeder is given support, a more positive feeding relationship can be established.

Promoting Feeding Success: One Step at a Time

To focus their attention on eating, children with neuromuscular problems that affect feeding may need a quiet environment with few distracting elements. These children may have less control of their muscles when they are in highly stimulating environments, which can increase the work associated with eating. See Box 3.2 for guidance on modifying a child's feeding environment (9,16).

Box 3.2   Guidelines for Child's Feeding Environment

- Child is comfortable and feels safe.
- Feeder can focus attention on child.
- Noise level in the room is not distracting.
- Items that distract the child from eating (eg, television and toys) are minimized.
- Temperature of the room is comfortable.
- Lighting is adequate.

Source: Data are from reference 9 and 16.

Clinical Tips

School cafeterias, which are usually noisy, may be too distracting for children with attention problems who have to concentrate on eating. Children need social interaction, so add a later snack if they were too distracted to eat enough at lunch. For some children who are easily distracted, however, eating lunch in the classroom with a small group may be more successful.

Generally, side-lying and prone positioning for eating should be discouraged because the alignment of the head and body may change the child's ability to control the jaw, tongue, and swallowing. Lack of stable jaw prevents the lips and tongue from operating from a stable, secure base. Box 3.3 provides information on modifying feeding positions (9,16).

Box 3.3   Guidelines for Optimal Feeding Position

- Head is midline.
- Head is tilted down and the neck is not extended.
- Sitting balance is stable and supported if necessary.
- Knees are bent.
- Feet are supported.

Source: Data are from references 9 and 16.

Clinical Tips

Specific feeding equipment for eating and positioning is needed both at home and school for some children with oral-motor feeding problems (1,6). If possible, confirm that the needed equipment is available and used at school.

Feeding is successful when the caregiver attends to the child's rhythm and signals of hunger and satiety, works to calm him or her, and develops mechanics of feeding that are effective with the child's particular emotional makeup, skill, and limitations. See Box 3.4, Box 3.5, and Box 3.6 for practical suggestions to maximize the feeding time.

Box 3.4   Feeding Tips for Caregivers

- Face the child to make eye contact at his or her level.
- Try to keep the level of anxiety about eating low.
- Set a comfortable pace and length for the meal.
- Smile and praise the child for small successful steps.
- Identify positive attention-seeking behaviors and respond with attention; this behavior may not be related to hunger. (Examples of positive behaviors include the child establishing eye contact and smiling, the child smacking lips after a taste, or the child attempting to name foods.)
- Ignore negative attention-seeking behaviors. (Examples of negative behaviors include dropping food to the floor or throwing it, kicking the table, whining.).
- Try to be consistent; avoid both overreacting and underreacting.
- Read nonverbal as well as verbal signs from the child.
- Do not use food as a reward; positive attention is a better reward.
- Seek support for feelings of anger, sadness, or frustration at mealtimes.

Box 3.5   Food Presentation Tips

- Small servings
- Foods that are separate rather than mixed
- Mild temperatures
- Bright colors (attract interest)
- Bland flavors (for infants)
- Sharper, spicier flavors (for older children)

Box 3.6   Suggestions for Scheduling Meals

- Regular structured time for meals, snacks, bed, and naps is necessary for most children.
- Most children will not eat if overly tired.
- Most children with congestion will eat less in the morning when congestion is worse.
- Children need snacks; five to six meals and snacks per day are common for young children.

Clinical Tips

Feeding therapy requires time just like any other behavior change. Some families work on feeding for a while and then stop. Leave the door open to try the therapy again, as the family's coping abilities permit.

Often a child with a special health care need will have a change in feeding as an early sign of another problem, just like children without special needs. An illness or a new staff member at school may explain a change in appetite.

Each family has its own "comfort foods" that are associated with fun and caring. Try to incorporate these foods into feeding interventions to make feeding and eating a positive experience for the family.

Referral for Feeding Problems

It is important to refer a child to a specialty interdisciplinary team for assistance with feeding and eating problems as soon as it is clear that these problems are beyond the usual level of difficulties. There are many messages in our society that equate successful feeding with being a good parent. A mother of a child with special needs and feeding problems may feel incompetent when well-meaning relatives and friends suggest they could get the child to eat. A parent who is frustrated, angry, and feeling unsuccessful in caring for a child is likely to be considered noncompliant, but simply may need additional support. Frustration of the child and parent from lack of progress in feeding and eating will delay more effective interventions that could be identified by a feeding team.

Feeding problems associated with child behavior and parent-child interaction may develop in children with oral-motor disorders as greater emphasis is placed on eating and meeting nutrition needs (2). It is often difficult to distinguish between physical, behavioral, and interaction problems. An interdisciplinary team approach is often more helpful (17). See Box 3.7 for services provided from specialty feeding teams (17–19).

Caregivers and children can benefit from behavior-modification programs. By learning how to identify interactive difficulties or tense situations related to food, dietetics professionals, public health nurses, and therapists often can intervene early and prevent full-blown behavior problems. See Box 3.8 for examples of feeding team interventions (18,19).

To summarize, children with special health care needs are at an increased risk of encountering feeding difficulties. To promote successful growth, families should be observant of the child's eating patterns. When feedings become stressful as a result of battling with the child to consume a meal, professional

Box 3.7   Specialty Feeding Teams

Potential Team Members
- Dietetics professional
- Speech-language pathologist
- Occupational therapist
- Physical therapist
- Nurse
- Social worker
- Pediatric gastroenterologist
- Developmental pediatrician
- Radiologist
- Psychologist or behavioral specialist

Services Provided
- Observe eating or feeding to assess and make recommendations for improving oral feeding.
- Order appropriate tests such as the modified barium swallow to confirm that oral feeding is safe.
- Assess nutritional status and growth and provide interventions.
- Assess for behavior-based feeding difficulties and provide therapy.
- Assist families in structuring meal and snack times and the feeding environment in the home.
- Recommend appropriate oral-feeding methods to stimulate oral-skill development.
- Coordinate related services such as wheelchair modifications or other positioning devices or equipment for self-feeding.
- Monitor intervention therapies at schools or programs to maximize skills.
- Follow-up with the child over time to assess growth and progress in developing feeding skills.

Ways to Access a Feeding Team
- Through the local early intervention program or special education department of the school system
- Through a pediatric hospital or facility with pediatric specialties
- Contact a local health department or other community programs with services for high-risk infants and children with special health care needs.

Source: Data are from references 17–19.

Box 3.8   Feeding Team Interventions—Examples

- Proper positioning during feeding, with home and school devices prescribed by appropriate physicians and related providers
- Special feeding techniques and utensils such as scoop plates or built-up spoons for self-feeding
- Specific food textures and consistencies for stimulating oral-motor sensations and chewing
- Energy goals plus meal and snack schedules for behavior and attention problems that interfere with eating
- Nutrient density and consistency changes to maximize oral-motor skills and decrease fatigue
- Oral-motor therapy techniques outside mealtime for some problems such as proprioceptive integration
- Referral for proprioceptive or neurophysiologic approaches as appropriate
- Therapy for specific oral-motor problems, such as muscle relaxation techniques for the upper lip
- Identify and support positive parent-child feeding interactions
- Parenting education or family counseling, as appropriate
- Additional diagnostic tests and medical interventions such as medications to reduce salivary gland secretions

Source: Data are from references 18 and 19.

---

assistance should be sought to assess the situation. Feeding difficulties do not have to consume the daily life of the child and family members. Feeding can become manageable when families seek the support of interdisciplinary team members.

Clinical Tip

Children with feeding problems are unlikely to "outgrow" primitive or abnormal behavior patterns without intervention. Specific therapy with a pediatric occupational therapist, physical therapist, or speech and language pathologist is needed as part of, or in addition to, the feeding team.

Case Examples

Example 1

Patient
A nonambulatory 18-month-old boy with poor muscle tone.

Problem
Child cries and chokes after swallowing only a few bites of oatmeal, grits, or other soft-textured foods. Mother is frustrated.

Findings
The boy is still being bottle-fed; PediaSure (Ross Products, Columbus, OH 43215) has been prescribed for weight gain. He is generally fed in his mother's arms. He was treated with medication for GERD and has increased his intake of PediaSure since treatment. There has been no increase in acceptance of foods by spoon. However, he self-feeds corn curls and vanilla wafers without choking. His mother is receiving inappropriate advice from relatives and is being told that she is "spoiling" the child.

Recommendations
- Reassure mother that her child is indeed hard to feed.
- Suggest placing the boy in his car seat to assure correct position for feeding.
- Refer the boy to a specialty feeding team for an evaluation of his resistance to texture in foods.

Rationale
GERD is documented in the child's history, and his poor muscle tone puts him at risk for aspiration. These factors must be evaluated before the feeding difficulty can be labeled a behavior problem, which is suggested by his ability to self-feed favorite foods without choking. If the problem is behavioral, an early intervention program or a feeding team with a behavioral specialist may be appropriate.

Example 2

Patient
A 2-year-old girl who was born at 32 weeks' gestation and is small for her age in weight and height for corrected age.

Problem
Eating position is on beanbag chair in front of the television.

Findings

The young, single mother is frustrated with suggestions that she feed her daughter more food. The mother considers the growth problem to be caused by her daughter's prematurity and, thus, unsolvable. The girl has a short attention span and is constantly on the go. Three generations, a total of six people, live together in one house. The grandmother thinks the girl needs discipline. The mother believes that her child will eat when she needs to and likes that the girl is entertained by the television.

Recommendations

- Assure the mother that her daughter's growth problem can be solved.
- Ask the mother to feed her daughter in the kitchen to minimize distractions. Suggest that the girl be seated at the table in a booster seat with a lap belt. This will ensure proper eating position and also keep the child from being able to constantly come and go.
- Recommend that only the mother and daughter be in the kitchen during mealtime initially; transition to scheduled family mealtimes when possible.
- Advise the mother to look at and praise her daughter for paying attention to her eating.
- Problem-solve with the mother to develop a regular meal and snack schedule.

Rationale

The findings of a lack of structured meal pattern and the ease with which the child is distracted from her eating indicate a behavior-based feeding problem. The 2-year-old is not likely to focus her attention on eating and chewing unless the feeding position is stable and the environment is conducive to eating. The young mother may need some support in parenting skills so that she is able to identify what is typical behavior for a 2-year-old.

Example 3

Patient

A 4-year-old boy who is overweight.

Problem

The child wants to eat all the time, even if he has just finished a meal.

Findings

The child is above the 95th percentile for body mass index–for-age; he is relatively sedentary. His favorite activity is sitting on the floor playing with his miniature cars. His family is relieved that he is eating because he was difficult to feed as an infant and was a picky eater as a toddler. The family attributes his difficult behavior to his age.

Recommendations

- The health care provider and the family should work out a structured meal and snack plan with some behavioral controls for restricting the boy's access to food.
- Advise the family to increase the boy's activity (eg, riding his tricycle outside or taking him to a park to play). Recommend that the boy be praised when he is more active.
- Try a behavior-modification plan for a short time, focusing on one target food or activity behavior; then reassess (ie, 1 month).
- Referral for further evaluation may be necessary, depending on the progress made during the trial.

Rationale

This overeating pattern can be seen in children who have experienced chronic illness or when food has been offered and accepted as a source of comfort. Refer for medical and psychological evaluation if the structured meal and snack plan and increased activity are not effective. Do not allow too much time to lapse before reassessing, because a more complete medical work-up is warranted if satiety cues fail to appear.

Example 4

Patient

A 3-year-old child who has a history of seizures.

Problem

The child has maintained the same weight for 6 months.

Findings

The child shows a decreased interest in eating. Seizure pattern has remained the same—one seizure per month. The child is on medications that are monitored every 3 months. The parents are now separated and the mother seems sad and anxious about her child and her situation in general. The dietary assessment of the child's eating showed an adequate variety of foods being offered and an appropriate meal pattern.

Recommendations

- Advise the mother on ways to increase the energy density of the child's food.

- Assess the potential effects of the anticonvulsant medication on appetite; consider a change in the timing of medication and meals.
- Consider a mother-child interaction problem; consider referring the mother to a mental health support professional.
- Consult with a pediatric neurologist if interest in food does not return after mother-child interaction improves.

Rationale

The mother may be depressed and need some counseling to deal with her own problems. The medications that the child is receiving to control the seizures may put the child at nutritional risk. The child's special health care need does not account for the presentation of eating problems as much as the typical reaction of a child to family disruption or maternal depression.

Example 5

Patient

A 6-year-old boy with a history of pulmonary problems.

Problem

Child resists eating food that does not have a soft, easy-to-chew texture.

Findings

The child was born prematurely and experienced bronchopulmonary dysplasia. The family rarely used child-care and kept the child at home away from germs and illnesses that could be contracted from other children. His parents consider it appropriate for him to eat casseroles, pasta, and other easy-to-chew foods. The boy has an individualized education program (IEP) that includes occupational therapy for development of fine motor skills. The boy's mother is requesting that the school lunch be modified to meet her son's likes, dislikes, and texture preferences. His teacher is using behavioral intervention when he frequently gets upset and has tantrums.

Recommendations

- Clarify the boy's developmental level; determine if he behaves more like a younger child because of his cognitive level or because of his inexperience interacting with other children.
- Refer for feeding evaluation by a feeding therapist or feeding team to determine oral-motor, sensory, and/or behavioral basis for food preferences.
- Provide feeding therapy and/or behavior intervention for the boy and his family, with focus depending on the outcome of the feeding evaluation.

Rationale

It is likely that the boy's feeding and eating problems have become behavioral, although they probably had medical and psychological bases originally. This type of problem is frequently seen in children with chronic diseases who may have had more opportunity than their age-matched peers to become manipulative with eating. If the boy has mental retardation, his picky eating habits and tantrums may also be consistent with his developmental level. If his cognitive level is typical, behavior management will be appropriate in the feeding area, as well as in other areas of concern. Unless there are documented nutrition or medical conditions warranting a modified school lunch, it is unlikely that a modified meal could be justified. However, the boy's IEP should include goals to address the feeding problem and expand his acceptance of foods and textures.

References

1. Morris SE. *Pre-feeding Skills: A Comprehensive Resource for Feeding Development.* Tucson, Ariz: Therapy Skill Builders; 1997.

2. Nardella M, Campo L, Ogata B, eds. *Nutrition Interventions for Children With Special Health Care Needs.* Olympia, Wash: Washington State Department of Health; 2002.

3. Barnard, K. *NCAST Feeding Scale.* Seattle, Wash: NCAST Publications, University of Washington School of Nursing; 1994.

4. Pipes PL, Glass R. Nutrition and special health care needs. In: Trahms CM, Pipes PL, eds. *Nutrition in Infancy and Childhood.* 6th ed. Columbus, Ohio: WCN/McGraw-Hill; 1997:377–405.

5. Anderson DM. Nutrition for premature infants. In: Samour PQ, Helm KK, Lang CE. *Handbook of Pediatric Nutrition.* 2nd ed. Gaithersburg, Md: Aspen Publishers; 1999:43–63.

6. Dunn M, Delaney T. *Feeding and Nutrition for the Child with Special Health Needs.* Tucson, Ariz: Therapy Skill Builders; 1994.

7. Carlson S, Armentrout C. *Neonatal Nutrition Handbook.* Iowa City, Iowa: University of Iowa Hospitals and Clinics Dietary Department; 1994.

8. *Feeding Management of a Child With a Handicap: A Guide for Professionals.* Knoxville, Tenn: University of Tennessee; 1990.

9. Howard RB, Winter HS. *Nutrition and Feeding Infants and Toddlers.* Boston, Mass: Little Brown and Co; 1994.

10. Carroll A, Garrison M, Christakis D. A systematic review of nonpharmacological and nonsurgical therapies for gastroesophageal reflux in infants. *Arch Pediatr Adolesc Med.* 2002;152:109–113.

11. Zerzan J, Glass R. Evaluating the young child who presents with growth concerns and feeding difficulties. *Nutrition Focus.* 1996;11(2):1–8.

12. Department of Nutrition and Food Service. *Pediatric Nutrition Handbook.* 3rd ed. Boston, Mass: Children's Hospital; 1993.

13. Lowman DK, Murphy SM, Snell ME. *The Educator's Guide to Feeding Children With Disabilities.* Baltimore, Md: Paul H Brookes Publishing Co; 1998.

14. Feucht S. Thickening foods for children. *Nutrition Focus.* 2003;18(5):1–6.

15. Pronsky ZM, Powers DE. *Powers and Moore's Food Medication Interactions.* 11th ed. Birchrunville, Pa: Food-Medication Interactions; 2000.

16. Taylor S, Wheeler LC, Taylor JR. Nutrition: an issue of concern for children with disabilities. *Nurse Practitioner.* 1996;21(10):17–18,20.

17. Wodarski LA. An interdisciplinary nutrition assessment and intervention protocol for children with disabilities. *J Am Diet Assoc.* 1990;90:1563–1568.

18. Hendricks K, Walker W. *Manual of Pediatric Nutrition.* 3rd ed. Philadelphia, Pa: BC Decker Inc; 2000.

19. Ekvall S. *Pediatric Nutrition in Chronic Diseases and Developmental Disorders: Prevention, Assessment, and Treatment.* New York: Oxford University Press; 1993.

Chapter 4

Non-oral Enteral Feeding

Janet Sugarman Isaacs, PhD, RD

N utrition support is required if oral eating and adequate growth cannot be assured. Nutrition support that uses the gastrointestinal tract is called enteral feeding and is the subject of this chapter. Children who are enterally fed completely by non-oral routes and those with some oral intake are discussed. Non-oral feeding may be required for a short or long time, and take place in homes and community settings. Non-oral feeding systems have various nicknames such as "tube," "g-tube," or "button" that reflect differences in practice sites. Gastrostomy feeding is the term used in this chapter to cover whatever devices are used for feeding directly into the stomach. This chapter does not cover nutrition support routes that do not use the gastrointestinal tract, such as total parenteral nutrition, or specialized modular components administered into the blood stream.

Difficult Family Decision

Feeding a child is an expression of loving parenting. Being unable to feed children so that they grow and thrive can undermine feelings of competence in parents (1). Most parents resist recommendations for gastrostomy placement or tube feedings in children of any age. After the newborn period, parents have been the main feeders and non-oral routes seem to take away their control of feeding their child. The family may need time to accept that non-oral feeding is necessary. Giving parents reasons why gastrostomy feeding will benefit their child coupled with affirmations for the parents may help them with the emotional coping required. The timing of the gastrostomy placement decision needs to be right. Delaying the decision too long raises risks for complications in a child with malnutrition. Rushing the parents into the decision may result in little cooperation and inadequate use of the feeding support system. Discussing the idea of nutrition support early, before it may be needed, can help families later when faced with the need for it. Family support groups are often helpful when discussing gastrostomy placement (see listing of Web sites at the end of the chapter).

Non-oral Feeding Devices and Specialty Feeding Teams

Types of non-oral feeding devices are the same in children with special health care needs (CSHCN) as for adult patients. Many conditions and diagnoses result in recommendations for non-oral feeding, as a result of undernutrition, aspiration, and risks related to coordination of breathing and eating (2). Diagnoses that require prolonged hospitalizations, are degenerative, or have a neurological component routinely involve non-oral eating. In some disorders, such as spastic quadriplegia, the need for non-oral nutrition support evolves over time, and in others, such as facial malformations, the need is seen early on and may lessen over time.

Table 4.1 describes the various feeding delivery systems covered in this chapter (3). (See Chapter 3 for a list of the types of providers and services that are needed to determine if non-oral feeding is necessary.) Specialty feeding teams are recommended especially for families who are entering the diagnostic process. Often families are reluctant to travel to find such a team, but coordinated, comprehensive care is more likely found in teams at major pediatric centers.

Table 4.2 identifies the signs and symptoms that indicate the need for nutrition support and specialty feeding teams (1,2). Box 4.1 and Table 4.3 provide examples of short- and long-term nutrition support. The most common type of gastrostomy placement is called a "PEG" which is percutaneous endoscopic gastrostomy (3,4). This laparoscopic surgery is generally a one-day or short hospital stay procedure. Gastrointestinal functional testing is routinely ordered prior to gastrostomy placement and usually can be done on an outpatient basis (5).

Clinical Tips

Pediatric specialists best manage pediatric gastrostomy placements and devices. Practitioners used to working with nursing homes or adults should be careful not to extrapolate from one group to another.

Specialty feeding teams are highly recommended for working with non-oral feeding issues. (See Chapter 3.) Community nutritionists should participate on the feeding team, or at least coordinate with the team as much as possible.

Table 4.1

Non-oral Feeding in Children With Special Health Care Needs

Type	Rationale/Example
Transpyloric feedings are through a tube from the nose or mouth into the upper part of the small intestine and are used short-term.	Infants and children with neurological disabilities have less sphincter tone in the lower esophagus and a higher risk of aspiration of stomach contents. Tube placement must be checked often to confirm its placement, so short-term use is likely.
Nasogastric or orogastric feedings go through a tube from the nose or mouth into the stomach and are used short-term.	Children with recent surgery or cystic fibrosis in which the discomfort of the tube is minimized by its short-term use or frequent removal and replacement.
Gastrostomy feedings go directly into the stomach through a device surgically placed through the abdominal wall, without additional surgery on the stomach or esophagus, for short- or long-term use.	Children who need to gain weight and who have normal gastrointestinal function test results, such as a child with a renal disorder or repaired diaphragmatic hernia.
Gastrostomy feedings go directly into the stomach through a device surgically placed through the abdominal wall, with additional surgery (fundoplication) to minimize stomach contents from backing up into the esophagus, generally for long-term use.	Children with abnormal gastrointestinal function tests, such as a risk for aspiration from spastic quadriplegia and swallowing coordination problems.

Source: Data are from reference 3.

What Goes into the Tube?

Feeding tubes have such a small diameter that only liquid nutrition is recommended. Everything that could obstruct or clog tubes must be avoided. Liquid forms of medications are recommended instead of crushed pills. Commercial complete nutritional supplements, an intermittent feeding pump, and related supplies such as bags and tubing are recommended for long-term users (5). Requirements such as letters of medical necessity and periodic prescriptions are routine for insurance coverage and provision of home health care agency services. Box 4.2 lists examples of products that are ordered for home nutrition support. Other formulas included in Chapter 2 Table 2.17 may be administered by tube.

Table 4.2
Signs and Symptoms Requiring Consideration of Non-oral Feedings

Signs and Symptoms in the Child	Signs and Symptoms Reported by the Family
• Inability to consume at least 80% of estimated energy needs or 90% of fluid needs by mouth • Indicators of malnutrition from lab work, anthropometric measurements, and growth history • Repeated unexplained upper-airway infections or pneumonia • History of GERD and failed medical treatment • History of weight loss or plateau with illness or surgery that does not correct with attempts at oral feeding	• Prolonged feeding times per meal or over the day • Frustration with feeding/eating; no longer a fun or positive way to interact with the child • Stopping the meal due to the child's choking, crying, and coughing as signs of discomfort • Hearing a "wet cough" after feeding or other signs of aspiration • Change of skin color, retching, vomiting, or other signs of distress with feeding or eating

Abbreviation: GERD, gastroesophageal reflux disease.
Source: Data are from references 1 and 2.

Box 4.1 Indications for Feeding Directly into the Stomach or Small Intestine (eg, Nasogastric, Nasoduodenal, or Nasojejunal Feeding)

- Recovery from an acute illness, during an exacerbation of a chronic condition such as cystic fibrosis, or for pre- or postsurgery periods when appetite or medications interfere with eating or when surgery impacts the oral structures.
- Unexplained failure to thrive without a suspected risk of aspiration.
- Malnourishment to the degree that the surgical risk for poor wound healing is too high to proceed with gastrostomy placement surgery.
- To rule out inadequate intake as a cause for weight loss, especially with behavioral problems such as frequent food refusal.
- Delay in initiating gastrostomy placement is required. An example may be the family that needs time to accept how acquired brain damage has affected feeding.

Table 4.3
Conditions Indicating Feeding By Gastrostomy

Diagnosis	Nutrition and Feeding Conditions
• Static encephalopathy or other central nervous system damage that causes risk of aspiration • Pierre-Robin or other congenital disorders associated with tracheomalacia • Tracheo-esophageal fistula, stricture, blockage, or other anomalies that interfere with the upper gastrointestinal tract • Severe spastic quadriplegia in which there is a risk or proven aspiration • Chronic kidney or liver diseases in which loss of appetite is common • Diaphragmatic hernia repair, gastochisis, or other anomaly of the digestive tract • Failure to thrive with failed oral feeding • Cystic fibrosis or other conditions that require high energy intake	• Muscle weakness in oral structures, which interfere with chewing and increase fatigue while eating • Poor muscle coordination of oral structures and swallowing so that there is a risk of aspiration • Food texture resistance with decreased energy intake over time • Weight loss over time with failed oral nutrition interventions • Loss of appetite or inability to respond to hunger cues • Negative associations with the mouth due to long-term pulmonary or cardiac disease that required respiratory support • Negative associations with the mouth that have resulted in oral hypersensitivity that causes gagging

Families without adequate insurance for costly supplies and formulas may want to prepare a homemade formula. Sanitation teaching and providing a specific recipe may work for short-term use, but homemade formulas are generally not recommended. Blending uncooked table foods, selecting foods based on taste rather than nutritional content, and underestimating fluid needs are common problems when homemade formulas are used. If there is no pump for night feeding, then all supplemental feedings have to be bolus fed during the day.

Management of Non-oral Feeding or Limited Oral Feeding

Box 4.3 describes services needed for implementing and monitoring non-oral feeding over time. The best intervention for a child who may require nutrition support is to refer the child to a specialty feeding team, or if this is not available, refer to a pediatrician or a pediatric gastroenterologist. The risk of aspiration with feeding requires evaluation, particularly in children with neurological

---

Box 4.2   Supplements and Formulas for Partial or Complete Gastrostomy Feeding

- Pediatric versions of complete nutritional supplements, such as PediaSure, Kindercal, Nutren Jr (1 kcal/mL; recommended for children 1 to 10 years of age)
- Adult complete nutritional supplements, such as Ensure (1 kcal/mL), for children older than 10 years
- Enrichment of beverages, such as Carnation Instant Breakfast added to milk (requires that cow's milk is tolerated)
- Partially digested formula with amino acids and medium-chain fatty acids, such as Peptamen Junior, for conditions in which intestinal absorption may be impaired
- Special formulas for inborn errors of metabolism, such as Propimex-2
- High-calorie booster for cystic fibrosis, such as Scandishake (may be concentrated to 2.5 kcal/mL in small volume for rare situations)

Pediasure, Ensure, and Propimex-2: Ross Products, Columbus, OH 43215; Kindercal: Mead Johnson Nutritionals, Evansville, IN 47721; Nutren Jr, Carnation Instant Breakfast, and Peptamen Junior: Nestlé USA, Glendale, CA 91203; Scandishake: SHS, Gaithersburg, MD 20884.

Box 4.3   Interventions for Non-oral and Limited Oral Feedings

- Assist the family with obtaining feeding equipment, supplies, and formulas.
- Assist the family in identifying community and specialty care providers.
- Help the family prepare for emergencies by troubleshooting ahead of time.
- Monitor the child's growth and set realistic weight goals aligned with the overall treatment plan.
- Adjust the schedule and volume as needed within the diet prescription for growth over time.
- Educate the family about potential tube feeding complications and how to prevent them.
- Identify signs and symptoms that would require referral back to the specialty feeding team or other specialist so the family can recognize a significant change that requires re-evaluation.

impairments. These children have a higher risk of aspiration due to gastrointestinal dysfunction, such as gastroesophageal reflux disease (GERD) and slow gastric emptying (6). A medical evaluation must determine if behavioral approaches for feeding intervention are safe.

Children with behaviorally based feeding problems such as refusing textures rarely require non-oral nutrition support. Yet they may benefit from the recommendations of team members for specific feeding interventions. Certain conditions, such as some inborn errors of metabolism, result in anorexia for which gastrostomy placement is recommended rather than behavioral interventions (7).

Schedules

After the need for nutrition support has been shown, close monitoring is needed to adjust goals and schedules over time. Table 4.4 provides examples of various goals in nutrition care plans. The continuum of care plans span from all to none for use of a gastrostomy for feedings. Reserving the gastrostomy for medications, meeting fluid needs, or only for sick days may be appropriate for some children, whereas others may require the gastrostomy for all medications and nutrition. The schedule must be based on the safety and sanitation of the formula being administered, such as hang times that consider contamination risks (8).

Any oral feeding that is safe should be encouraged for socialization and education planning. Even if the amount of oral feeding that the child enjoys is small, it is worth maintaining in the feeding schedule. The family's input into the feeding schedule that best fits their home life is recommended.

When long-term gastrostomy feeding is planned, bolus feedings during the day can be timed to fit the meal and snack schedule of the family or school (1). When a return to oral feeding is a long-term goal, daytime bolus feedings without night feedings may make it less likely this goal can be reached. Frequent daytime bolus feedings may lower the hunger sensation and interest in oral feeding over time. Offering oral foods or beverages before bolus feedings may encourage interest in tasting, but maintaining oral hunger sensations is difficult with closely spaced eating or bolus feeding times.

Goals for growth and feeding skill progression and the overall medical condition are individualized to the child. Tables 4.5 and 4.6 are examples of monitoring and trouble-shooting that allow reassessment of the nutrition care plan for a child. Complications of enteral feedings, such as gastrointestinal, malabsorption, nausea and vomiting, fluid/electrolyte, and mechanical should be referred to the medical provider or the dietetics professional working with the family (2).

Table 4.4
Goals and Schedules for Non-oral and Limited Oral Feedings

Goal	Schedule Example
Weight gain is the primary goal, with a secondary goal of maintaining oral eating.	More than half of estimated energy needs are provided at night by pump feedings, with an oral lunch, supper, and snack during the day.
Progressing oral feeding skill development is the primary goal, with a secondary goal of weight gain.	Three meals and two snacks are offered during the day, with bolus feedings by gastrostomy provided after meals or at night based on the energy deficit from the day's oral intake.
Recovery from recent illness and regression in feeding skills.	80% of total needs provided by night feedings and bolus feedings during the day, with oral tastes of favorite foods as much as tolerated.
Transition off gastrostomy feeding is the primary goal, with a secondary goal of weight maintenance (with medical clearance).	Reduce night feedings by 25% and omit some bolus feedings during the day to allow hunger sensations to emerge; offer frequent snacks during the day.

Table 4.5
Monitoring Gastrostomy Feedings

Assessing Fluid Volume and Schedule	Questions for the Caregiver/Family
• What product is going into the gastrostomy or nasogastric tube? • How many milliliters or fluid oz per feedings? • What times are the bolus feedings? • How long does a bolus feeding take? • Are you using a feeding pump at night? • How many bolus feedings per day? • How much water is used to flush the tube each feeding? • Does the child seem comfortable after the feeding? • How do you tell if the child is hungry? • Do you think this feeding schedule fits the school and family routine?	• Do you have any problems with the gastrostomy site? • Do you see signs of constipation or diarrhea? • Does the child vomit or attempt to vomit when he or she is not sick? • What are the instructions if this button needs replacing? (Or if the balloon breaks? Or for replacing the nasogastric tube?) • Do you or your relatives think your child's weight is about right? (Or too low or too high, as appropriate.) • Do you have any problems getting the formula? • Do you sometimes have to turn off the pump during the night? • What other people are able to feed your child in addition to yourself?

Clinical Tips

The goal for the child's eating may change over time, based on the family's emotional and coping style rather than the child's diagnoses.

Insurance, schools or programs, and funding sources can pose limitations that affect the progression of eating or feeding skills; for example the funding source may pay for the nutritional supplement to go into the gastrostomy tube but not into the mouth. See Table 6.6 in Chapter 6 for possible reimbursement sources for nutrition products and services.

Table 4.6
Management of Gastrostomy-Related Problems

Problem	Suggestions for Management
Rapid weight gain or rate faster than expected for age.	Reduce kcal/kg/day by reducing rate or time of feedings while maintaining adequate fluid volume.
Constipation or decrease in stooling on a liquid diet.	Switch to a fiber-containing complete nutritional supplement and confirm that adequate fluids are given.
A parent thinks the child is missing the taste of food and the mouth is dry.	If swallowing is safe, oral tastes can be encouraged. If swallowing is not safe, wet lips often with oral gel or water.
Gastrostomy site is oozing, inflamed, or uncomfortable.	Routine medical visits are needed to size the device correctly and to have medications prescribed for granulation tissue.
Child is pulling on device or tubing.	Adjust clothing or netting to cover the abdomen area; do not restrict use of hands.

Returning to Oral Feeding

Returning to oral feeding after non-oral feeding may or may not be a reasonable goal. It is best to proceed slowly and balance non-oral and oral intake with other therapeutic and family priorities (1). Table 4.7 provides signs of readiness to return to regular eating. Transition times vary greatly, and require school involvement, community service providers, and financial sources for providing formulas (9). Ideally, the child's nutritional status should stay stable as the transition occurs. Continued involvement of a specialty feeding team is vital, par-

---

Clinical Tips

- If the child is dependent in care and must be lifted and transferred, the family may prefer the child to stay the same weight even if weight gain is recommended. The weight issue may be a sign of their concerns about the future for their child in general. Health professionals should discuss the importance of overall good health and nutritional status for the child, and help the family identify physical and mechanical resources to deal with lifting and transferring.
- Families of a child who require nutrition support generally have had a lot of frustration about oral eating in the past. The assumption that eating is fun and a social activity for the family may not apply.
- If a child has a gastrostomy (or nasogastric tube) and is also allowed oral eating, the nutritional adequacy of the oral food may not be as important as its texture and consistency in maintaining or progressing oral feeding skills.
- As the child gains weight, the gastrostomy button may need to be changed to a different length or diameter. If the hole is getting bigger, the device is sized incorrectly and more leakage is likely.

---

ticularly because behavioral consultation may be required. The transition process removes some of the control of feeding from the parents and medical providers and places more control with the child. Often, a sign that the transition is successful and gastrostomy feeding is no longer needed is the child eating well after an illness passes.

Long-Term Nutrition Support: Assessment and Evaluation

Children with chronic illness for whom oral feeding is not a safe option need to have nutrition support evaluated routinely over time. Table 4.8 illustrates conditions in which long-term gastrostomy feeding is typical. Depending on age and the medical condition, the energy, protein, and micronutrients being fed need to be assessed quarterly, or at a frequency ordered by the child's primary care providers.

Scoliosis that develops over time may change the stomach emptying time and activity level. Medication adjustments can change growth and nutrient requirements. Common problem nutrients are calcium and phosphorus, which may be inadequate in low-calorie and low-protein diets. Standard nutrition recommendations based on age and gender usually overestimate needs for gastrostomy-fed

Table 4.7
Management of Returning to Oral Feeding

Signs of Readiness for a Successful Transition	Roles for Community Providers
• Child has interest in oral eating and wants to taste. • The family can identify signs of hunger in the child. • Child is at a healthy weight and could tolerate a small weight loss. • Family support and interest for working on oral feeding is assured. • A school or therapy program is involved with the plan and has staff with feeding expertise. • Medical evaluation has ruled out risk of aspiration. • A transition-feeding plan has been developed with follow-up care identified.	• Assist the family in identifying subtle signs of hunger. • Develop a plan to decrease the frequency of bolus feedings or adjust the feeding schedule to leave a block of at least 3 hours for hunger sensations to be stimulated. • Recommend attractive and easy-to-eat foods for oral stimulation and tasting. • Monitor the child's weight and growth. • Monitor the child's fluid intake as the volume of nutritional supplement is reduced. • Offer family support for continuing oral feedings after food refusals or behavioral problems.

Table 4.8
Long-Term Gastrostomy Feeding: Examples of Nutrition Plans

Condition	Example of Nutrition Care Plan
7-year-old girl with spastic quadri-plegia and seizures, with no sitting balance.	• Two bolus feedings per day and 10 hours/night on pump with extra water flushes when medications given • Providing adequate energy and protein intake from a complete pediatric product, based on her size and level of activity.
4-year-old boy with propionic acidemia (an inborn error of protein metabolism) with age-appropriate eating skills, and hospitalizations about two or three times per year.	• A low-protein diet of table foods and beverages, with gastrostomy feeding of his metabolic formula when his oral intake is less than required, when he needs extra fluids, or for formula and medications when ill.
5-year-old girl with Rett syndrome who is unable to gain weight.	• Three meals and two snacks per day fed orally with night gastrostomy feedings for extra energy and nutrients from a complete nutritional supplement.
8-year-old boy with glycogen storage disease (an inborn error of carbohydrate metabolism) who and eats and drinks normally.	• Night gastrostomy feeding to prevent hypoglycemia and preserve growth. Regular foods and beverages (as allowed on his low-sugar diet) are offered as frequent meals and snacks during the day.

children who are stable with a chronic condition. Formulas that are selected for the child at the time of gastrostomy placement should be reevaluated to adjust for energy density, calcium, phosphorus, fiber, and other nutrients (2,10). Although parents should have input into the feeding schedule, the composition, rate, and fluid needs for the child should be determined and updated by the medical provider and dietetics professional.

Case Examples

Example 1

Patient
A nonambulatory 23-month-old boy with low muscle tone.

Problem
Need for feeding re-evaluation.

Findings
His mother is frustrated because he cries and chokes after swallowing only a few bites of oatmeal, grits, or other soft-texture food. His referral to feeding intervention through his early intervention program has resulted in a change of his feeding position at home, a meal and snack schedule, and consistent behavioral rewards for trying textures. His mother is stressed by his lack of progress and two episodes of chest congestion and bronchitis in the last 4 months. He was previously treated for GERD and has increased his volume of PediaSure (Ross Products, Columbus, OH 43215) since treatment, but has not improved in accepting food from a spoon. His weight and length are about the same over the last 5 months due to his illnesses, according to his mother.

Recommendations
Reassure the mother that her child is hard to feed, and refer them to a specialty feeding team for his texture resistance. His upper respiratory illnesses may be linked to his therapy, so continuing feeding intervention work with him is not recommended. Specific swallowing studies and gastric emptying studies may be needed to clarify his gastrointestinal dysfunction.

Rationale
A behavioral basis for his feeding problems has been ruled out for now and further medical evaluation is required. His underlying neurological disability puts him at continued risk of aspiration that must be reevaluated. Surgical or medical interventions need to be considered because feeding interventions have been tried and have not been effective.

Example 2

Patient

A nonambulatory 3-year-old girl with high muscle tone (hypertonicity or spasticity).

Problem

Need for non-oral feeding support.

Findings

She has a history of weight loss with frequent illness, with only part of the weight regained. The girl's body mass index (BMI) and triceps skinfold fat mass are less than the 5th percentile for age. The family is pushing her to eat a high-fat, energy-dense diet with three meals and three snacks offered per day. The girl is refusing to eat by pushing the food away and crying, which progresses to vomiting about once per week. The family is frustrated by her crying and poor sleeping schedule. They have offered favorite foods and drinks at night in their efforts to increase energy intake. She is more irritable than she used to be. The family is concerned because orthopedic surgery could be scheduled if she would stay well.

Recommendations

Reassure the family that their child is hard to feed, and refer them to a specialty feeding team for comprehensive feeding evaluation and intervention to correct failure to thrive with failed oral refeeding.

Rationale

There is sufficient evidence of chronic undernutrition from her frequent illness, low fat stores, and body weight to suggest that malnutrition is likely. Her irritability and sleep problems may be possible signs of her low nutritional reserves and hunger. The need for a long-term gastrostomy may be avoided if she gets transpyloric feeding for a short time. If the child and family are too frustrated by this negative feeding experience, she may lose oral skills over time if a gastrostomy is required. The nutritional problem should be addressed prior to orthopedic surgery.

Example 3

Patient

A nonambulatory 7-year-old boy who had a gastrostomy placed at age 5.5 years for failure to thrive and severe oral-motor feeding problems.

Problem
Possible rapid weight gain over the last year.

Findings
The family tells nutrition professionals and medical providers how much easier their life is now that he has been gastrostomy fed compared with the terrible time they had trying to get him to eat. Their friends thought he would die because he was so small and thin before. The child is administered a complete nutritional supplement by night feedings and by three bolus feeding during the day, with oral tastes as he tolerates. His family has noticed he likes cookies and ice cream at night. At school he is getting therapy for spoon-feeding. The school reports he eats about one third of his meal, which is more than the family sees him eat at home.

He has gained almost 5 kg and about 3 cm in height over the last 18 months, but is below the fifth percentile for height, and at the 10th to 25th percentile for weight. His height is estimated by recumbent length due to his scoliosis, so his BMI may not be a valid indicator. His triceps skinfold measurement on his dominant arm is between the 50th and 85th percentile. His scoliosis brace has been outgrown, and his wheelchair is requiring adjustment. His mother is delighted about his increased weight and hopes he gains more because others in her family are large.

Recommendations
Determine if the family has been in touch with the specialty providers about his feeding schedule and volume, which needs to be adjusted for his current status. Coordinate with the team to decrease the daytime bolus feedings and also the night feeding rate to decrease his total energy intake to prevent overweight, and encourage oral feeding at home and school. The mother is still reacting to her feelings of frustration when he was failing to thrive, and needs support to understand that he may not grow to be as tall as other family members but could become too fat.

Rationale
There is sufficient evidence of overweight from his triceps skinfolds to decrease his energy intake from his gastrostomy feedings in a step-wise fashion. His scoliosis invalidates conclusions from his height and BMI. The issue of transitioning off gastrostomy feeding could be considered in the future if the family can move past his early negative oral feeding experiences. The child's ability to progress in his self-feeding skills is encouraging, but does not yet predict if he will signal hunger and fullness successfully enough to maintain a healthy weight.

Example 4

Patient

A nonambulatory 8-year-old boy with cerebral palsy who had a gastrostomy placed for failure to thrive and severe oral-motor feeding problems when he was 5 years old.

Problem

Weight plateau over the last year.

Findings

His weight has stayed the same even though the specialty feeding team increased the bolus volume about 6 months ago. His recumbent length was used to estimate his stature, which is the same as last year. The child has had a decrease in triceps skinfolds fat mass on his dominant arm to the 15th percentile. (His fat mass on that same arm was closer to the 50th percentile for his age when measured 6 months ago.) His school provided physical therapy last year but he did not make much progress. He is dependent in his care. He cannot participate by bearing weight on his legs when being transferred. The family has no problem getting the formula and the gastrostomy site is clean and dry. His mother does not consider his lack of weight gain a problem and quoted a local physician who told her all children with cerebral palsy were small.

Recommendations

Determine his current intake, including formula, volume, and feeding schedule. Review the priorities that the family has for their son with a focus on concerns for lifting and transferring him. Once a good rapport is established, ask whether weight gain would be acceptable to them. Even if they are not concerned about his size, suggest that they may want to be sure he is getting sufficient fluids so that he is comfortable and avoids constipation.

Rationale

The family may have been unwilling to challenge the authority of the specialty providers in the goal for weight gain, and are skipping bolus feedings or shutting off the night feeding pump. Their main concerns may be his long-term care, and their inability to afford a bigger wheelchair, lift him into the bathtub, or some back problem in a parent. Once such concerns are identified, community resources can generally address them.

References

1. Morris SE, Klein MD. *Pre-Feeding Skills: A Resource for Comprehensive Mealtime Development.* 2nd ed. Therapy Skill Builders. Harcourt Health Sciences Co; 2000.
2. Pediatric enteral support. In: Nevin-Folino NL, ed. *Pediatric Manual of Clinical Dietetics.* 2nd ed. Chicago, Ill: American Dietetic Association; 2003:471–493.
3. Levy SE, O'Rourke M. Technological assistance innovations for independence. In: Batshaw ML, ed. *Children with Disabilities.* 5th ed. Baltimore, Md: Paul H. Brookes; 2002:637–639.
4. Effects of gastrostomy feeding in children with cerebral palsy: an AACPDM evidence report. May 2002. Available at: http://*www.aacpdm.org*. Accessed October 25, 2003.
5. Staiano A. Food refusal in toddlers with chronic diseases. *J Pediatr Gastroenterol Nutr.* 2003;37:225–227.
6. Sandritter T. Gastroesophageal reflux disease in infants and children. *J Pediatr Health Care.* 2003;17:198–205.
7. Batshaw ML, Tuchman M. PKU and other inborn errors of metabolism. In: Batshaw ML, ed. *Children with Disabilities.* 5th ed. Baltimore, Md: Paul H. Brookes; 2002:333–345.
8. Bott L. Contamination of gastrostomy feeding systems in children in a home-based enteral nutrition program. *J Pediatr Gastroentol.* 2001;33:266–270.
9. Schwartz SM, Corredor J, Fisher-Medina J. Diagnosis and treatment of feeding disorders in children with developmental disabilities. *Pediatrics.* 2001;108:671–676.
10. Institute of Medicine. *Dietary Reference Intakes for Energy, Carbohydrate, Fiber, Fat, Fatty Acids, Cholesterol, Protein, and Amino Acids.* Washington, DC: National Academy Press; 2002. Available at: http://www.nap.edu. Accessed March 4, 2004.

Additional Resources for Parents and Professionals

Exceptional Parent Magazine (http://www.eparent.com)

Federal Interagency Coordinating Council Site for Families with Children with Disabilities (for finding local intervention programs) (http://www.fed-icc.org)

Federation for Children with Special Needs (http://www.fcsn.org)

National Information Center for Children and Youth with Disabilities (targeted mainly toward educational programs) (http://www.NICHCY.org)

National Organization for Rare Diseases (NORD) (http://www.rarediseases.org)

Chapter 5

Fluid and Bowel Problems

Janet Sugarman Isaacs, PhD, RD

C hildren with special health care needs (CSHCN) have the same problems with fluid and bowel management as other children, but encounter these problems more often. Families frequently mention fluid and bowel management problems when asked what their child eats and drinks. Parents may select specific foods and beverages based on their concerns or beliefs about constipation, diarrhea, or fluid needs. Some chronic health conditions result in key symptoms, such as the characteristic smell of urine in maple syrup urine disease or floating stools in celiac disease. Some chronic conditions are sensitive to fluid balance and can worsen with low fluid intakes that may not stress a healthy child. Fluid and bowel problems require interventions appropriate to the age and chronic condition of the child.

Normal Bowel Function and Fluid Needs

Normal patterns of bowel function clearly are different than constipation and diarrhea in healthy infants and children, and families recognize constipation and diarrhea as signs of possible acute gastrointestinal upset. In children with special health care needs, constipation and diarrhea can occur due to gastrointestinal reasons, but also from medication side effects, overall muscle tone, or a reaction to stress. Common patterns of bowel movements are detailed in Table 5.1 (1). Tables 5.2 and 5.3 identify common causes of constipation and diarrhea (2,3).

Constipation in healthy children may be linked to inadequate dietary fiber intake. Fiber recommendations from the dietary reference intakes (DRIs) for children are based on 14 g of dietary fiber per 1,000 kcal consumed (4). (For further information, refer to Chapter 2.) For a 4- to 8-year-old child, 25 g of dietary fiber is recommended (4). These recommendations are more than the "age + 5 grams" previously recommended for children older than 2 years. For some children with special health care needs, it may be difficult to achieve the DRI for

Table 5.1

Usual Bowel Function in Infants and Children

Bowel Movements in Infants	Bowel Movements in Children

• Exclusively breastfed infants have more frequent and looser stools than bottle-fed infants.
• Bottle-fed infants:
  • 4–5 bowel movements per day in week 1 of life
  • 2 bowel movements per day before solid foods introduced
  • After introduction of solid foods: < 2 bowel movements per day
	• Age 1–3 y: 1–2 bowel movement per day
	• > 3 y: 1 bowel movement per day
	• Toddler's diarrhea is a common type of loose stool with strong and sudden urge to defecate shortly after a meal.
	• Stool retention and straining is commonly a part of toilet training.

Source: Data are from reference 1.

Table 5.2

Causes of Constipation in Healthy Infants and Children

Non-Nutritional Causes	Nutrition-Related Causes
• Fever • Infections or other concurrent illness • Sudden major change such as starting school or taking a vacation • Toilet training • Inappropriate use of laxatives • Medications	• Decrease in dietary fiber intake • Decreased fluid intake with weaning • Pica or other non-food ingestion • Food allergy • Iron supplements

Source: Data are from references 2 and 3.

Table 5.3

Causes of Diarrhea in Healthy Infants and Children

Non-Nutritional Causes	Nutrition-Related Causes
• Fever • Infections or other concurrent illness • Sudden major change, such as starting school or taking a vacation • Inappropriate use of laxatives • Medications	• Excessive intake of apple or other fruit juice • Increase in intake of dietary fiber • Pica or other non-food ingestion • Food poisoning • Food allergy • Beverages or foods with sugar alcohol (such as sorbitol)

Source: Data are from references 2 and 3.

Clinical Tips

- In infants and children, constipation, diarrhea, and vomiting are common responses to any illness, and frequently the cause cannot be identified.
- Families ascribe food allergies and intolerance as causes of constipation and diarrhea more commonly than can be medically documented.
- Functional constipation in toilet training is a common result of the child consciously withholding stool and may require a medical as well as nutritional approach.

Clinical Tip

Some high-fiber foods, such as popcorn, peanuts, and raisins, can be choking hazards and should not be offered to young children or children with oral-motor feeding difficulties.

fiber, and total energy intake should be considered. There are no recommendations for dietary fiber for infants (4).

Because bowel problems are closely related to overall fluid balance, Table 5.4 provides fluid needs for various ages and weights (2,3). Box 5.1 and Box 5.2 illustrate how to assess the adequacy of fluid intake in healthy infants and children and when the assessment should result in referral to medical care.

Clinical Tips

- A "rule-of-thumb" is that excessive formula intake for infants is considered to be > 32 fluid ounces per day, especially if the infant is younger than 5 months and solid foods have not been started.
- After solid foods are begun (at 4 to 6 months), up to 32 fluid ounces of formula per day is typical, and additional fluids such as water and juice diluted with water may be supplemented.
- Excessive fluid intake in children tends to replace more nutritious solid foods and may result in a total intake low in iron, fiber, and other nutrients.
- Low fluid intake for infants younger than 5 months and not yet on solid foods may result in inadequate energy intake for growth.

Table 5.4
Fluid Needs

	Fluid Needs
Infants	
Healthy, weight < 10 kg	80–120 mL/kg
Premature	Use healthy infant fluid needs and consult with specialty care providers for special conditions such as bronchopulmonary dysplasia, in which fluid may be increased or decreased.
Children	
Weight < 10 kg	80–120 mL/kg
Weight > 10 kg	1500–3000 mL/m^2

Daily Fluid Recommendations by Weight of Child	
Weight, kg (lb)	**Recommendation**
3.2 (7)	2 cups (16 fl oz, 480 mL)
5.5 (12)	3–3.5 cups (24 fl oz, 720 mL)
9.5 (21)	5 cups (40 fl oz, 1200 mL)
11.8 (26)	6 cups (48 fl oz, 1440 mL)
16.4 (36)	7 cups (56 fl oz, 1680 mL)
20 (44)	8 cups (64 fl oz, 1920 mL)

Source: Data are from references 2 and 3.

Box 5.1   Assessment of Fluid Intake

- Is there low fluid volume for age?
- Is there excessive fluid volume? Is there water craving such as excessively drinking bath water?
- Are fluids self-restricted to one or two types?
- Is there choking on liquids?
- Are thicker liquids such as milkshakes handled with less difficulty than thin liquids, such as water?
- Are typical drinks delivering caffeine or iron-binders, such as sweet tea?

Box 5.2   Fluid Problems Requiring Medical Referral

- Diarrhea—watery bowel movements every 1 or 2 hours. Dehydration may develop and require oral rehydration therapy
- Chronic diarrhea (> 2 weeks) or acute diarrhea (< 2 weeks) that has not been evaluated
- Refusal to eat or drink, unexplained fever, unexplained vomiting as signs of acute illness
- Concentrated urine
- Increased thirst (ongoing), water craving, or excessive water intake, such as drinking bath water

---

Assessment of CSHCN

Nutritional and Non-nutritional Causes of Constipation and Dehydration

The underlying condition may be a more likely basis for constipation and fluid management problems than dietary choices in children with special health care needs. Table 5.5 (1,2) and Boxes 5.3 and 5.4 identify conditions and diagnoses in which constipation and dehydration are likely, and whether they are related to dietary intake.

The usual dietary recommendations for fiber, fluids, and exercise must be adjusted for the child's condition, use of over-the-counter products, and prescribed medications. Laxative doses and the frequency of their use may account for both diarrhea and constipation. If blood is visible in stools or the child experiences abdominal distension or pain, medical attention is needed immediately (1,2). Obstipation or impaction is usually treated with laxatives or enemas and then a home management program (3).

Clinical Tips

- The muscles on the inside of the body may work the same as those on outside of the body. If a child has little voluntary control of their large muscle movements, such as in spastic quadriplegia, it is likely that they will have problems with constipation based on the involuntary muscle movements in the gastrointestinal track.
- Because seizures and dehydration seem to be related, children who have seizures may be at greater risk if their fluid intake is low. Dehydration is an early sign of a concurrent illness.

Table 5.5

Causes of Constipation and Diarrhea in CSHCN

Constipation	Diarrhea
Non-nutritional causes	
• Decreased motor activities due to impaired mobility and fewer position changes • Abnormal muscle tone impacts colon motility • Medications that impact muscle tone or cause nausea • Neurological disability or diagnosis such as shunt blockage • Nonambulatory status • Damage to sacral nerves or spine • Drugs that slow peristalsis	• Fecal impaction or blockage • Medications such as antibiotics that result in changes in intestinal flora • Change in CNS, particularly in degenerative conditions
Nutrition-related causes	
• Low-texture foods provide low dietary fiber • Feeding position that limits fluid intake • Oral-motor feeding problems • Low volume or rate of gastrostomy feeding	• High-fiber foods • Too much juice • Fast feeding rate that results in dumping-type problems • Volume or rate changes in gastrostomy feedings • Lactose intolerance after acute illness

Abbreviations: CNS, central nervous system; CSHCN, children with special health care needs.
Source: Data are from references 1 and 2.

Box 5.3   Conditions Associated with Constipation in Children With Special Health Care Needs

- Anal stenosis or fissures
- Medications that slow peristalsis
- Encopresis
- Hirschsprung's disease
- Anatomical defect
- Myotonic dystrophy
- Spastic quadriplegia
- Spina bifida
- Static encephalopathy
- Down syndrome

Box 5.4   Conditions Associated With Dehydration in Children With Special Health Care Needs

---

- Oral-motor feeding difficulties, especially with drooling
- Short bowel syndrome or ileostomy
- Condition with prescribed diuretics such as cardiac conditions or bronchopulmonary dysplasia
- Seizures with post-ictal state, poorly controlled
- Inability to signal thirst

Fluid and Bowel Management for CSHCN

Providing medical nutrition therapy by increasing fluids and dietary fiber can be effective for mild fluid and bowel problems in CSHCN. However, signs and symptoms of fluid imbalance or the start of constipation are subtle. For example, loss of appetite in a nonverbal child may be a key sign of constipation.

Excessive intake of juices or other high-sugar drinks may cause diarrhea. These are not recommended as a treatment of dehydration or management of diarrhea (5). For healthy children ages 1 to 6 years, guidelines for juice intake of 4 to 6 fluid ounces per day are an appropriate starting point for children with special needs (5). See Chapter 2 for more on juice intake. Conditions in which high carbohydrate intakes are required are rare, such as inborn errors of protein metabolism.

Management of constipation and ways to add dietary fiber and increase fluids are described in Tables 5.6 and Box 5.5 (2). Keep in mind that fluid and constipation problems can progress to medical emergencies in vulnerable children. Immediate referral back to the child's pediatrician, specialty health care team, or emergency service is appropriate for some children. Children who should be referred include those with a history of dehydration or fluid overload for pulmonary or cardiac problems requiring prescribed medications such as furosemide (Lasix). Children with a history of impaction or possible signs of impaction should be referred for medical evaluation and management.

Medications

Be sure to check prescribed medications for possible food and drug interactions and for side effects including diarrhea and constipation (1). Box 5.6 identifies some of these medications. Adding medications or physician-approved over-the-counter products to manage the constipation is often necessary for constipation

Table 5.6

Constipation Management

Constipation Problem	Intervention	Typical Patient
Intermittent	• Increase dietary fiber and confirm adequate fluid intake	• Ambulatory child with mental retardation
Chronic, with gas and abdominal pain, no medical attention required	• Increase dietary fiber and fluid intake • Increase physical activity • Use of laxatives if physician recommends	• Child with Down syndrome • Child with little ambulation resulting from hemiplegia
Chronic, as above, with anal fissure or pain on evacuation	• Physician visit • Low-dose laxative • Dietary modifications as ordered by physician	• Child with spastic quadriplegia
Chronic, with loss of appetite and cramping, no relief with over-the-counter remedies	• Physician visit • Educate about risks of enemas and prescribed laxatives • Dietary modifications as ordered by physician	• Older nonambulatory child with scoliosis • Child with prescribed medications for seizures and for pain from hip dislocation

Source: Data are from reference 2.

Clinical Tips

- If a child is already on a regimen of chronic laxatives, dietary fiber modifications are not likely to be effective. At most, they may allow reducing the daily laxative dose required.
- Try to avoid offering mineral oil as a lubricant at mealtimes, although absorption of fat-soluble vitamins from foods consumed with mineral oil may not be decreased significantly.
- Managing constipation as a chronic condition is often necessary and is more effective than treating one episode at a time.
- Corn syrup (eg, Karo) may be effective for some children. Depending on the amount used, it may contribute a significant amount of energy. Corn syrup should not be used for infants due to the risk of botulism.
- Add dietary fiber gradually to avoid uncomfortable symptoms of gas and bloating as the intestinal flora change. Make sure water is encouraged to prevent constipation from the increased stool volume.

Box 5.5   Bowel Management by Dietary Fiber and Fluids

- Increase foods derived from plants:
  - Whole-wheat bread and crackers
  - Oatmeal and oat bran breads and cereals
  - Cereals containing fiber (such as those containing 3 g dietary fiber/serving)
  - Fresh fruits and vegetables, such as an apple with peel
  - Beans such as kidney, northern, or navy, lentils
  - Sweet or white potato with skin
- Decrease foods that do not provide dietary fiber (to level of nutritional adequacy):
  - White bread
  - Meats
  - Macaroni and cheese
  - Beverages with low percentage of fruit juices, carbonated beverages
  - Puddings and other dairy-based products, if calcium intake is adequate
- Identify the fiber content of processed foods from food labels, and select those with a high level of fiber.
- Identify the fiber in complete nutritional supplements, if used, and select the higher fiber version.
- Increase fluid intake by adding liquid snacks between meals. Water is the preferred liquid unless other goals such as weight gain are involved. If non-oral feeding is used, increase the volume used to flush before and after tube feeding.
- Establish a toileting routine or schedule in coordination with the child's school or program.
- Discuss toileting "accidents" and the social consequences of soiling and/or cost of diapers with the family and child and provide or refer for support services as needed.
- Identify the child's level of activity or exercise, and increase activity if feasible, considering the child's positioning needs and physical abilities.
- Confirm that the family has discussed prescribed medications, over-the-counter bulking laxatives, enemas, and clean-out procedures with the medical care providers or assess whether referral to a specialty team is needed.
- Confirm that the family understands gastrointestinal function sufficiently to notice early signs and symptoms of dehydration and bowel impaction.

Source: Data are from reference 2.

Box 5.6   Medication Groups Associated With Constipation

Anesthetics and some pain medications
Analgesics (eg, Tylenol-3)
Anticonvulsants (seizure medications)
Antidepressants (may be used also for behavioral management)
Antispasticity drugs (eg, Baclofen)
Barium
Ferrous sulfates and other medications for iron repletion of blood

---

management. Table 5.7 identifies types of prescription and over-the-counter laxatives (1,6).

Increasing Fluids for Infants and Children

Increasing fluids may be necessary to avoid dehydration as a result of acute losses from diarrhea, vomiting, and fever as shown in Table 5.8 (7,8). For some CSHCN with feeding difficulties, fluid intake is low because liquids are more difficult to handle in the mouth and can cause choking. Fluid and electrolyte changes can impact many neurological conditions such as shunted hydrocephalus and seizure medication levels. Prevention of dehydration is a part of good care even in terminal illness and in palliative care (9).

Oral rehydration therapy (ORT) or intravenous fluids may be medically necessary if early signs of needing fluids are not identified (8,10). Nutritional approaches must be coordinated with the child's specialty care or primary care physician. Refer infants with special health care needs to their primary physician or specialty physician if formula or breastmilk intake is so low that increasing fluid intake is required. It is currently recommended to continue formula or breastmilk through an episode of diarrhea (8,11). If there is a need for an electrolyte-containing fluid such as Pedialyte (Ross Products, Columbus, OH 43215) in place of breastmilk or formula, refer to the child's physician (12).

Case Examples

Example 1

Patient
A nonambulatory 18-month-old boy with low muscle tone.

Table 5.7

Commonly Used Bowel Management Products and Laxatives

Agent	Generic Examples (Brand Names)*	Mechanism of Action	Side Effects
Osmotics	• Lactulose • Polyethylene glycol (Miralax) • Sorbitol • Barley malt extract • Magnesium hydroxide (Milk of Magnesia) • Magnesium citrate	Draws water into intestine resulting in distention and peristalsis	Cramping, flatulence, risk of magnesium poisoning in infants. Magnesium overdose can unbalance electrolytes and minerals.
Lubricant	• Mineral oil	Softens stool and decreases water absorption from intestine	Anal leakage, risk of aspiration
Stimulant	• Senna (Senokot) • Bisacodyl • Glycerin suppositories	Increased intestinal motility	Abdominal pain, rare case reports of shock-like reactions
Emollient	• Docusate (Colace)	Softens stool by mixing in water and fat	For short-term use only
Bulk-forming	• Psyllium fiber (Metamucil) • Calcium polycarbophil (FiberCon)	Adds insoluble fiber to increase distention and peristalsis	Abdominal pain, blockage

*Miralax, Braintree Laboratories, Braintree, MA 02185; Milk of Magnesia, Bayer Healthcare, Morristown, NJ 07962; Senokot and Colace, Purdue Pharma, Stamford, CT 06901; Metamucil: Procter & Gamble, Cincinnati, OH 45202; FiberCon, Wyeth Consumer Healthcare, Madison, NJ 07940.

Source: Data are from references 1 and 6.

Table 5.8
Increasing Fluid Intake

Need	Intervention	Typical Patient
Increase fluids to cover losses from vomiting; acute illness	• Offer typical foods on regular diet but add water, strained fruit juices, gelatin, Popsicles, clear bouillon, or broth. • Electrolyte-replacement drinks (eg, Pedialyte*) may be physician-ordered for specific situations.	• Previously healthy child with an acute illness
Increase fluids after an acute illness if the child refuses to accept solid foods; regression in feeding skills	• A full-liquid diet includes milk and milk-based products, and blended or pureed foods made into a liquid. • Commercially produced complete nutritional supplements are appropriate if required long term. • Electrolyte-replacement drinks (eg, Pedialyte*) may be physician-ordered for specific situations.	• Child with Down syndrome • Child with oral-motor feeding problems who fatigues with eating • Child with a history of prematurity and frequent pulmonary infections
Increase fluids after an illness in which gastrointestinal sensitivity is noted by cramping and low appetite with re-feeding.	• Commercially produced complete nutritional supplements are appropriate as slow return to usual foods is likely. • A low-residue diet is not recommended. It is too restrictive for long-term use.	• Child with spastic quadriplegia • Child recovering from surgery • Child with a change in seizure pattern and medication
Increase in fluids due to low intake of all foods and refusal to drink.	• If no new oral problems are noted, consider a feeding evaluation and swallowing studies to assure safety and to assess if non-oral feeding is required for fluids needs.	• Nonambulatory child • Child with Rett syndrome

*Pedialyte, Ross Products, Columbus, OH 43215

Problem
Need for chronic constipation management.

Findings
His mother is attempting to wean him from a bottle. His daily fluid intake is reduced by approximately 8 fluid ounces in the transition to drinking from a cup. He likes to eat a low-texture diet. He had episodes of refusing to eat and periods of infrequent hard stools during his first year.

Recommendations
Consider constipation management as part of his neuromuscular disability, and try a two-pronged approach: dietary intervention by encouraging fluids and increasing fiber, and management by use of a daily low-dose bulk laxative.

Rationale
Dietary methods alone are unlikely to be sufficient, and the goal is to avoid fecal impaction as a medical emergency or depression of appetite from chronic constipation. Intermittent treatment of constipation may have a worse outcome than routine prevention of constipation.

Example 2

Patient
A 28-month-old boy with oral-motor feeding difficulties.

Problem
Excessive fluid intake.

Findings
He prefers to drink liquids rather than eat solid foods. On previous days, fluid intake was 32 fluid ounces of whole milk, 12 fluid ounces of apple or grape juice, and 14 fluid ounces of a fruit-flavored drink. He refused breakfast and self-fed 6 french fries and less than one fourth of a cheese sandwich at lunch. The snack and supper intake were mostly refused, with less than half the offered serving consumed. Dietary analysis showed adequate energy but inadequate iron, fiber, and vitamins.

Recommendations
Fluids should be decreased to 28 fluid ounces of milk and 8 fluid ounces of juice per day with liquids mostly offered after meals and snacks have been eaten. Additional water may be given when thirsty. Fruit-flavored drinks, carbonated

beverages, and teas are used only as special treats and offered rarely, such as once every 2 weeks.

Rationale
The child finds the work of eating harder and maybe more fatiguing than drinking. Oral skills may improve with time and practice; so self-feeding and spoon-feeding are encouraged. High fluid needs may relate to drooling or oral losses while eating, but liquids should not replace more nutritionally dense foods. If oral skills are not sufficient to provide enjoyment at meals and snacks, a complete nutritional supplement may be needed in place of some meals.

Example 3

Patient
A 24-month-old boy with shunted hydrocephalus and an oral-motor feeding problem.

Problem
Constipation with a complete nutritional supplement.

Findings
He requires a complete nutritional supplement for 60% of total energy. Oral feedings are soft table foods, primarily fruits (applesauce, canned peaches) and starches (oatmeal and mashed potatoes). The mother, who noticed unexplained crying and infrequent bowel movements, considers constipation a problem. Over-the-counter constipation remedies were only effective for a short time.

Recommendations
Discontinue the over-the-counter products. Switch to the same nutritional supplement that has added dietary fiber. Over 3 to 4 days, transition to the fiber-containing complete nutritional supplement for 25%, then 50% of total volume of the supplement needed each day. Although some CSHCN do well with 100% of the fiber-containing supplement, adjusting the proportions of fiber-containing formula and regular formula for the individual child works best. Monitor to prevent diarrhea and do not change use of other medications during the introduction of the new formula. A fiber-containing supplement may not be needed long-term, depending on the types of table foods tolerated.

Rationale
Additional dietary fiber in the complete nutritional supplement offers more consistent constipation management than use of intermittent over-the-counter

remedies. Some children with neurodevelopmental disabilities respond well to additional dietary fiber in complete nutritional supplements. If this is not sufficient to prevent constipation, medical management rather than over-the-counter products may be required.

Example 4

Patient
A 3-year-old boy with shunted hydrocephalus and infrequent bowel movements.

Problem
New symptoms of fecal incontinence or suspected fecal impaction.

Findings
His mother thinks that he has abdominal cramps and a decreased appetite. Home remedies, such as prune juice and mineral oil, have been ineffective.

Recommendation
Refer to pediatrician or local emergency room.

Rationale
This could become a medical emergency due to the child's underlying diagnosis, even though shunt problems are unlikely.

Example 5

Patient
A 3-year-old girl with seizures.

Problem
Starting a new prescribed seizure medication coincides with onset of a constipation problem.

Findings
She has increased drowsiness, questionable nausea, and constipation. As a result, both food and fluid intake are reduced. The mother reported these symptoms to the prescribing physician who continued the current regimen for 2 more weeks.

Recommendations
Increase her fluid intake and call the physician to ask if over-the-counter laxatives will be appropriate to use. Make sure the mother knows how to replace

fluids lost due to vomiting and report signs of dehydration to the prescribing physician if they occur.

Rationale

This may not be routine constipation due to the child's underlying diagnosis, but perhaps may be a transitional drug side effect. Medical oversight is required, but the symptoms may disappear over 2 weeks when they go back for follow-up appointment. Temporary treatment of constipation and watchful waiting are good steps during this interim.

References

1. Baker SS, Liptak GS, Colletti RB, Croffie JM, Di Lorenzo C, Ector W, Nurko S. Constipation in infants and children: evaluation and treatment. A medical position statement of the North American Society for Pediatric Gastroenterology and Nutrition [errata in *J Pediatr Gastroenterol Nutr.* 2000;30:109]. *J Pediatr Gastroenterol Nutr.* 1999;29:612–626.

2. Nevin-Folino NL ed. *Pediatric Manual of Clinical Dietetics* 2nd ed. Chicago, Ill: American Dietetic Association; 2003.

3. Siberry GK, Iannone R. *The Johns Hopkins Hospital The Harriet Lane Handbook.* 15th ed. Philadelphia, Pa: Mosby Inc; 2000:229–256.

4. Institute of Medicine. *Dietary Reference Intakes for Energy, Carbohydrate, Fiber, Fat, Fatty Acids, Cholesterol, Protein, and Amino Acids.* Washington, DC: National Academy Press; 2002. Available at: http://www.nap.edu. Accessed March 4, 2004.

5. American Academy of Pediatrics. The use and misuse of fruit juice in pediatrics. *Pediatrics.* 2001;107:1210–1213.

6. Laxatives. Available at: http://www.healthsquare.com. Accessed March 4, 2004.

7. Tolboom JJ. Management of severe malnutrition and diarrhea. *J Pediatr Gastroenterol Nutr.* 2000;30:346–348.

8. Duggan C, Nurko S. "Feeding the gut": the scientific basis for continued enteral nutrition during acute diarrhea. *J Pediatr.* 1997;131:801–807.

9. Ethical and legal issues in nutrition, hydration, and feeding (position paper). *J Am Diet Assoc.* 2002;102:716–726.

10. Grandjean AC, Reimers KJ, Buyckx ME. Hydration: issues for the 21st century. *Nutr Rev.* 2003;61:261–271.

11. Farthing MJ. Oral rehydration: an evolving solution. *J Pediatr Gastroenterol Nutr.* 2002;34(Suppl 1):S64-S67.

12. Institute of Medicine. *Dietary Reference Intakes for Water, Potassium, Sodium, Chloride, and Sulfate.* Washington, DC: National Academy Press; 2004. Available at: http://www.nap.edu. Accessed March 4, 2004.

Chapter 6

Community Services and Programs

Janet Horsley Willis, MPH, RD

Identifying Needs

When working with children with special health care needs (CSHCN) and their families, it is important to identify programs in which they are participating and those to which they may be referred to access additional nutrition services. Eligibility requirements and program benefits vary from state to state for each program. Although many programs serve children of all ages, several are targeted for specific age groups. Table 6.1 provides a list of key questions to ask parents/guardians about their child's nutrition service needs and access to resources.

Community-Based Programs and Resources

Special Supplemental Nutrition Program for Women, Infants, and Children Referral Criteria

The Special Supplemental Nutrition Program for Women, Infants, and Children (WIC) is a federally funded community nutrition program targeting low-income pregnant and lactating women, infants, and young children up to age 5 years. Many low-income infants and children with special health care needs will qualify for WIC services (1). Contact your local health department for specific WIC eligibility requirements, and refer to Table 6.2 for general program information (1).

Early Intervention Programs

Early intervention programs are established through Part C of the Individuals with Disabilities Education Act (IDEA) to ensure that infants and toddlers with developmental disabilities have access at an early age to services and supports, including nutrition services. The early intervention services include interdisciplinary

Table 6.1

Identifying Nutrition Services and Product Needs

Infants and Toddlers, Birth to 3 y	Preschool-Age Children, 3–5 y	School-Age Children, >5 y	Questions to Ask: Does your child ...
X	X	X	Have a dietetics professional or nutritionist with whom you are working?
X	X	X	Need a special pediatric formula or diet?
X	X	X	Need special feeding equipment (ie, bottles, nipples, spoons, forks, plates, etc)?
X	X	X	Require tube feeding?
X	X		Participate in the WIC Program?
X			Participate in the Early Head Start Program?
X			Receive therapy services through an early intervention program and have an IFSP?
	X		Participate in the Head Start Program?
	X	X	Receive therapy services through school, and have an IEP or 504 accommodation plan?
X	X	X	Receive health services through a pediatric specialty clinic, Children with Special Health Care Needs Program, and/or Medicaid/Medical Assistance Program?

Abbreviations: IEP, individualized education program; IFSP, individualized family service plan; WIC, Special Supplemental Nutrition Program for Women, Infants, and Children.

evaluations, care coordination, special therapies for the child, and respite and support services for the family. Registered dietitians are considered personnel qualified to provide services for infants and toddlers in the early intervention system. Qualifications for registered dietitians are established by each state based on recommendations from the State Interagency Coordinating Council that provides oversight and sets policies for the service delivery system.

School-Based Nutrition Services

Many schools across the country participate in the National School Breakfast Program and National School Lunch Program, which provides balanced meals

Table 6.2
WIC Program Eligibility Criteria and Benefits

Eligibility Criteria	Program Benefits
• Income guidelines based on family size and gross annual income • Infants and children up to the age of 5 years • Nutrition risk factors including low iron levels, elevated serum lead levels, underweight, short stature, failure to thrive, obesity, premature birth or low birth weight, high-risk medical condition, inadequate diet, feeding delays, and environmental risks.	• Nutrition and health education • Nutrition assessments and evaluations • Food package that may be modified for CSHCN if a diet prescription is provided (eg, a special formula may be substituted with proper documentation)* • Monitoring of immunizations • Community referrals

Abbreviations: CSHCN, children with special health care needs; WIC, Special Supplemental Nutrition Program for Women, Infants, and Children.
*Allowances and requirements for modifications may vary from state to state.
Source: Data are from reference 1.

for school children. CSHCN should have equal access to these meal programs due to civil rights protections and supporting regulations from the US Department of Agriculture (USDA), which administers these meal programs (2). Based on federal guidelines, school meals are to be modified at no extra charge for a student whose medical condition restricts his/her diet and who has a diet prescription on file at the school. These modifications are required for children with disabilities. However, schools may make meal modifications at their discretion for individual children who do not have disabilities but who are medically certified as having a special dietary need (2).

Public and private schools that do not participate in the USDA—sponsored food and nutrition programs are not required to follow these specific guidelines. However, related legislation such as Section 504 of the Rehabilitation Act of 1973 and the Americans with Disabilities Act require that reasonable accommodations be provided for children with disabilities (3). School policies should provide information on meal modifications in these school settings.

The following information describes the allowable meal modifications following the USDA guidelines for the National School Breakfast Program and National School Lunch Program.

Diet Prescription for a Child with a Disability

Substitutions will be provided for a child with a disability only when supported by a diet prescription signed by a licensed physician (2). The prescription must include the following components:

- A statement of the child's disability and an explanation of why the disability restricts the diet
- A statement identifying the major life activity affected by the disability
- A list of foods to be omitted from the child's diet and the foods that may be substituted

Diet Prescription for a Child with a Chronic Condition

For a child who does not have a disability, but who has a chronic medical condition that requires a special diet, a prescription or medical statement must be signed by a recognized medical authority (ie, a physician, a physician's assistant, a nurse practitioner, or any other specialist identified by the state education agency) (2). This prescription must include the following components (also refer to Figure 6.1 [4]):

- A statement identifying the medical or other special need that restricts the child's diet
- A list of foods to be omitted from the child's diet and a list of the foods that may be substituted

Menu Modifications

Diet prescriptions may specify modifications of the school breakfast and lunch menus to accommodate specific children. Table 6.3 provides potential menu modifications for a low-calorie diet, high-calorie diet, and texture modifications: chopped, ground, and pureed (4).

Educational Program Goals and Objectives: Nutrition

The Americans with Disabilities Act of 1990 protects individuals with disabilities from discrimination and provides equal access to programs and services. Likewise, supportive state and federal legislation mandates education and related services for children with disabilities who enroll in public schools. The Individualized Family Service Plan (IFSP), Individualized Education Program

Diet Prescription for Meals at School

Name of student for whom special meals at school are requested:

_____

Disability or medical condition that requires the student have a special diet. Include a brief description of the major life activity affected by the student's disability.

_____

Diet Prescription (Check all that apply)

____ Diabetic   ____ Reduce Calorie

____ Increased Calorie   ____ Modified Texture

____ Other (describe) _____

Foods Omitted and Substitutions (Please check food groups to be omitted. List specific foods to be omitted and suggest substitutions using the back of this form or attach information.)

____ Meat and Meat Alternatives   ____ Milk Products

____ Bread and Cereal Products   ____ Fruits and Vegetables

Textures Allowed (Check the allowed texture.)

____ Regular   ____ Chopped   ____ Ground   ____ Pureed

Other information Regarding Diet or Feeding (Please provide additional information on the back of this form or attach to this form.)

I certify that the above named student needs special or school meals prepared as described above because of the student's disability or chronic medical condition.

_____
Physician/Recognized Medical Authority Signature   Office Phone Number   Date

Figure 6.1   Diet prescription for meals at school. Reprinted from *CARE: Special Nutrition for Kids*. Revised ed. Montgomery, Ala: Alabama State Department of Education, Child Nutrition Programs; 1995:21, with permission from Alabama State Department of Education.

Table 6.3

Sample Menu Modifications for School Breakfast and School Lunch

Breakfast Menu	Low-Calorie	High-Calorie	Chopped	Ground	Pureed
Orange juice	No change	No change, or substitute fruit nectar	No change	No change	No change; thicken with applesauce if needed
Oatmeal	Serve plain	Add margarine and powdered milk	No change	No change	May need to puree with milk, or replace with cream of wheat or grits
Cinnamon roll/butter	Replace with plain toast	Add margarine	Cut into bite-size pieces	Replace with more hot cereal or grits	Replace with more hot cereal or grits
Milk	Low-fat or fat-free	Whole	Whole, low-fat, or fat-free	Whole, low-fat, or fat-free	Whole, low-fat, or fat-free

Lunch Menu	Low-Calorie	High-Calorie	Chopped	Ground	Pureed
Hamburger	No change	Add cheese	Chop meat	Grind meat, add sour cream	Puree beef with broth or tomato soup
Buns	Serve plain	Add margarine	Cut into quarters or substitute noodles	Substitute rice or chopped noodles	Substitute bread crumbs mixed with the pureed beef, or pureed mashed potatoes
French fries	Baked potato	No change	Mashed potatoes	Mashed potatoes	Puree mashed potatoes and blend with gravy or milk
Broccoli	No change	Add margarine or cheese sauce	Well-cooked and chopped	Well-cooked and mashed	Pureed with cream soup

Lunch Menu	Low-Calorie	High-Calorie	Chopped	Ground	Pureed
Canned peaches	No change, if canned in own juice	No change, or canned in syrup or peach nectar	Cut into bite-size pieces	Chopped and mashed	Puree with juice or nectar
Milk	Low-fat or fat-free	Whole	Whole, low-fat, or fat-free	Whole, low-fat, or fat-free	Whole, low-fat, or fat-free

Source: Adapted from *CARE: Special Nutrition for Kids.* Revised ed. Montgomery, Ala: Alabama State Department of Education, Child Nutrition Programs; 1995:77–90, with permission from Alabama State Department of Education.

(IEP), and the 504 Accommodation Plan are working documents that secure services for CSHCN in educational programs. These individualized plans are developed for children who require specialized services in early intervention and public school—based programs. The IFSP is written for infants and toddlers up to age 3 years who have developmental disabilities and are being served in early intervention programs. The IEP is designed for preschool and school-aged children with disabilities to provide special education and related services that are appropriate for their learning needs. For school-aged children who are chronically ill and do not require special education services but who have special dietary issues, a 504 Accommodation Plan can be developed. Table 6.4 summarizes the educational programs and planning tools that are available for CSHCN in these settings.

Individualized plans include annual goals or outcomes, short-term objectives, and a schedule for evaluation. Parents, therapists, and staff are involved in the planning process to ensure that appropriate goals and objectives are identified and monitored for each child. Each goal and objective should be measurable so that the child's progress can be assessed within a designated time period. Incorporating nutrition goals and objectives into these plans will facilitate the delivery of services to improve the nutritional status of CSHCN (4–7). Table 6.5 provides an outline of program considerations for developing nutrition-related goals and objectives for an IFSP, IEP, or 504 Accommodation Plan (5). Examples of goals and objectives are provided in Boxes 6.1, 6.2, and 6.3.

Table 6.4

Educational Programs and Planning Tools for CSHCN

	Setting		
	Early Intervention Program	**Public School (Special Education)**	**Public School (No Special Education)**
Child	Infants and toddlers birth to 3 years with developmental disabilities	School-age children receiving special education services	School-age children with chronic conditions who do not require special education services
Criteria	Infants and toddlers who have a demonstrated delay in at least one of the following areas: cognitive development, physical development, language and speech development, psycho-social development, or self-help or adaptive skills; or have a diagnosed physical or mental condition that puts the child at high risk for developmental delays. Examples include seizure disorder, intraventricular hemorrhage, fetal alcohol syndrome, spina bifida, congenital or acquired hearing loss, visual impairment, genetic disorder, brain or spinal cord trauma, inborn errors of metabolism, microcephaly, failure to thrive, symptomatic congenital infection, etc.	Children with physical or mental disabilities that substantially limit one or more major life activity. Examples include autism, hearing and visual impairments, mental retardation, multiple disabilities, orthopedic impairment, other health impair-ment, emotional dis-turbance, specific learning disability, speech and language impairment, traumatic brain injury, etc.	Children with chronic conditions that may require health-related services, but do not require special education services. Examples may include chronic renal disease, controlled seizure disorder, cystic fibrosis, diabetes, hemophilia, juvenile arthritis, etc.
Planning tool	IFSP	IEP	504 Accommodation Plan

Abbreviations: CSHCN, children with special health care needs; IEP, Individualized Education Program; IFSP, Individualized Family Service Plan.

Clinical Tips

- When referring an infant or toddler to early intervention services, there must be a documented disability, a demonstrated delay in one or more domains (eg, cognitive, developmental, speech, motor, psychosocial, or self-help skills), or a diagnosis of a physical or mental condition that puts the child at high risk for developmental delays (refer to Table 6.4). Infants and children with special health needs may have feeding problems or altered energy needs that lead to failure to thrive (previously addressed in Chapter 2). For example, these feeding problems are often identified in premature and low-birth-weight infants, and young children with bronchopulmonary dysplasia, cerebral palsy, or Down syndrome. Failure to thrive is considered a physical condition that puts a child at risk for developmental delays and may provide a basis for enrollment in early intervention services. However, other nutritional deficits and growth delays are often difficult to quantify as part of the eligibility criteria for early intervention. To identify a child eligible for services, other health care providers or therapists may need to determine percent delays in one or more of the mentioned domains. Once enrolled in the early intervention services, a young child's nutrition and growth issues should be documented so that they are addressed in the care plan and integrated into the IFSP.
- Work with an interdisciplinary feeding team to address complex feeding problems in infants and children (previously addressed in Chapter 3).

Clinical Tips

- Work with parents/guardians to secure nutrition services in schools and early intervention programs by requesting a nutrition plan in the IFSP, IEP, or 504 Accommodation Plan. Encourage parents to request these additions to the plan and be available to provide consultation to the planning team.
- If you are working with a school-aged child who requires a special diet, ask about the child's participation in the school breakfast and lunch programs. Provide parents/guardians with a diet prescription if a menu modification or food substitution is required and contact the foodservice manager at the school.
- If a child requires a snack as part of his/her meal plan at school, it must be scheduled with the school. Snacks are not considered part of the standard school meal plan and are not provided by the Child Nutrition Program or other school program unless they are specified in the IEP or 504 Plan. Some families may decide to send snacks to school for their child.
- In addition to making provisions for meal modifications, continue to educate children about their nutrition so that they can learn to make healthful food choices. Encourage older children and adolescents to take responsibility for their diet and food choices.

Table 6.5
Nutrition Goals and Program Considerations

Nutrition Goals	Program Considerations
• Develop or refine self-feeding skills. • Improve mealtime behavior. • Communicate nutrition needs such as hunger or thirst. • Improve growth.	• Identify special feeding equipment and measuring equipment for tracking growth. • Identify supervision needed for mealtime. • Identify positive reinforcements for correct responses. • Identify personnel responsible for specific tasks such as tracking weight and growth measurements, providing scheduled snacks, monitoring progress on specific goals, etc. • Provide training for staff.

Source: Adapted with permission from Horsley JW, Allen ER, Daniel PW. *Nutrition Management of School Age Children With Special Needs: A Resource Manual for School Personnel, Families, and Health Professionals.* 2nd ed. Richmond, Va: Virginia Department of Education and Virginia Department of Health; 1996:57–58.

Box 6.1   Early Intervention Program Nutrition Plan

Patient:
A 20-month-old boy with Down syndrome and developmental delays.

JW receives physical therapy, occupational therapy, and nutrition services through the local early intervention program. He drinks fluids from a bottle and eats strained baby foods three times per day. In addition to his delayed feeding skills, he eats only a limited variety of foods. He has an Individualized Family Service Plan (IFSP) that includes a nutrition component.

IFSP Nutrition Goal/Outcome:
JW will demonstrate improved feeding skills.

IFSP Nutrition Objectives:
- JW will practice cup-drinking skills at one meal, 5 days per week for the next 3 months.
- JW will try at least one new food each week at home for 6 months.
- JW will progress to eating pureed foods without resistance at home and at the early intervention program within 6 months.

Box 6.2   School Nutrition Plan in Special Education

Patient:
A 7-year-old girl with spastic cerebral palsy and a seizure disorder.

SH is extremely underweight and has delayed feeding skills. Her lunch is pureed and an aide feeds her at mealtime. Her Individualized Education Program (IEP) includes a nutrition component to address her need for weight gain.

IEP Nutrition Goal:
SH will demonstrate improved weight gain and growth during the school year.

IEP Nutrition Objectives:
- SH will drink 4 oz of an energy-dense/high-protein supplement with her school breakfast 75% of the time.
- SH will eat a school lunch supplemented with energy-dense additives (ie, margarine, powdered milk, cheese sauces, gravy, etc) 75% of the time.

Box 6.3   School Nutrition Plan for a 504 Accommodation Plan

Patient:
A 9-year-old boy with type 1 diabetes mellitus.

BJ is in a regular education program with a 504 Accommodation Plan for his diabetes. He receives insulin injections, and his physician has prescribed a diabetic diet that is composed of three meals and three snacks daily. He is growing well. He needs supervision to ensure that he eats his snacks on a regular schedule to prevent episodes of hypoglycemia.

504 Plan Nutrition Goal:
BJ will maintain blood glucose levels within normal limits.

504 Nutrition Objectives:
- BJ will eat a snack at 10 a.m. and 2 p.m. on at least four out of five days at school.
- BJ will report his blood glucose levels to the school nurse every Friday morning with 90% compliance.

Reimbursement for Nutrition Services and Products

When developing the nutrition care plan for a CSHCN, it will be important to clarify reimbursement issues related to the following:

- Nutrition follow-up services
- Pediatric formula, supplements, and modular products
- Special feeding equipment
- Feeding tubes, pumps, and supplies

Refer to Table 6.6 to identify appropriate resources to provide these services and products.

Eligibility criteria and program benefits for these programs vary from state to state. Information may be obtained by contacting the programs in a locality, or checking Web sites for the state program on the Internet. For referral information, contact the local health department, school district, or department of social services in the community.

Parent Advocacy and Support Groups

In addition to offering emotional support, parent support groups and advocacy groups can help families with children who have special health care needs gather information and navigate the service system. Each community is different in how parents and patient advocacy groups are organized. The local telephone directory, library, and neighborhood newspapers are generally better sources than the national headquarters for locating a specific group. The Internet is a resource for finding information and locating other families of children with rare syndromes and disorders. Families and providers should be cautioned that nutrition misinformation and financial frauds may be mixed with credible information on the Internet and by local groups, so it is important to carefully review information and ask questions to validate the reliability of claims. Recommending groups for psychosocial support and encouraging parents to ask questions or bring materials to clinic appointments may help families obtain accurate information.

Internet Resources

To learn about programs from a national perspective, the Web sites listed in Box 6.4 may be useful. Keep in mind that there is variability in program criteria and benefits in every state.

Table 6.6

Possible Sources of Reimbursement for Nutrition Services, Formula and Special Feeding Equipment and Supplies

NOTE: Availability of formula, supplies and services, as well as eligibility criteria will vary from state to state.

Potential Funding Source	MNT	Pediatric Formula and Tube Feeding Products	Metabolic Formula for the Treatment of Inborn Errors of Metabolism	Tube Feeding Supplies*	Special Feeding Equipment[†]
Early Intervention Programs/IDEA: Part C	Registered dietitians who meet the minimum training criteria as specified by the State Personnel Preparation Committee, Interagency Co-ordinating Council, are qualified to provide and supervise early intervention services. They may be a part of the early intervention team or hired as consultants to provide services.	Potential payor of last resort for eligible children, particularly if specified in the IFSP.	Potential payor of last resort for eligible children, particularly if specified in the IFSP.	Potential payor of last resort for eligible children if specified in the IFSP.	Potential payor of last resort for eligible children, particularly if specified in the IFSP. Assistive Technology Program is a potential resource, as well.
Head Start and Early Head Start	Certain programs may have a dietetics professional or nutrition consultant; focus is	Must have a diet prescription on file with the meal modification, substitutions, or	Must have a diet prescription on file with the meal modification, substitutions, or	N/A	N/A

(continued)

Table 6.6 (*continued*)

Potential Funding Source	MNT	Pediatric Formula and Tube Feeding Products	Metabolic Formula for the Treatment of Inborn Errors of Metabolism	Tube Feeding Supplies*	Special Feeding Equipment[†]
Head Start and Early Head Start (*continued*)	usually on general nutrition education rather than specialized services. All children in the program receive nutrition services as a part of the federal guidelines.	additions, including special formula needs.	additions, including special formula needs.		
Indian Health Services	Potential resource for nutrition services for eligible families. Nutrition services may be arranged contractually or a referral may be made to the WIC Program for nutrition services, formula/ food package.	N/A	N/A	N/A	N/A

Table 6.6 *(continued)*

Potential Funding Source	MNT	Pediatric Formula and Tube Feeding Products	Metabolic Formula for the Treatment of Inborn Errors of Metabolism	Tube Feeding Supplies*	Special Feeding Equipment†
Medicaid/Medical Assistance: EPSDT Services and Medical Waiver Program	Potential payment mechanism for nutrition services; strict criteria for providers and numbers of visits.	Resource for families enrolled in Medicaid; criteria for formula provision varies by state.	Resource for families enrolled in Medicaid; formula provision varies by state.	Resource for families enrolled in Medicaid.	Potential payment mechanism for special feeding equipment.
Pharmaceutical companies and charitable organizations	N/A	Emergency supplies may be available for families in need.	Emergency supplies may be available for families in need.	Emergency supplies may be available for families in need.	Special bottles and nipples are available from certain companies for cleft lip/palate and neonatal units or nurseries.
Private insurance	Reimbursement for nutrition services varies; the dietetics professional must have a provider number to bill for services; check with your state MNT Reimbursement representative through the state dietetic association.	Formula coverage varies according to insurance company.	Formula coverage varies according to insurance company and state mandates.	Potential payment mechanism.	Coverage varies according to insurance company.

(continued)

Table 6.6 *(continued)*

Potential Funding Source	MNT	Pediatric Formula and Tube Feeding Products	Metabolic Formula for the Treatment of Inborn Errors of Metabolism	Tube Feeding Supplies*	Special Feeding Equipment†
SCHIP [States have different names for this program.]	Potential payment mechanism for nutrition services.	Resource for families enrolled in SCHIP; criteria for formula provision varies by state.	Resource for families enrolled in SCHIP; formula provision varies by state.	Resource for families enrolled in SCHIP.	Potential payment mechanism for special feeding equipment.
State Title V: CSHCN Program	Potential source of nutrition services or payment mechanism.	Potential payment mechanism as a last resort for eligible children.	Potential payment mechanism as part of state metabolic treatment program.	Potential payment mechanism as a last resort for eligible children.	Potential payment mechanism as a last resort for eligible children.
SSI Note: SSI eligibility may also assist a child to be eligible for Medicaid (see Medicaid section).	Monthly cash payment may be used to pay for nutrition services; SSI eligibility may also assist a child to obtain Medicaid as another avenue for nutrition services reimbursement (see Medicaid Section).	Monthly cash payment for eligible children may be used to purchase formula.	Monthly cash payment for eligible children may be used to purchase formula or special foods.	Monthly cash payment for eligible children may be used to purchase tube feeding supplies.	Monthly cash payment for eligible children may be used to purchase feeding equipment.
TRICARE/ CHAMPUS (insurance coverage for military families)	Potential payment mechanism for nutrition services for eligible families.	Potential resource for eligible families.	Potential resource for eligible families.	Potential resource for eligible families.	Potential resource for eligible families.

Table 6.6 *(continued)*

Potential Funding Source	MNT	Pediatric Formula and Tube Feeding Products	Metabolic Formula for the Treatment of Inborn Errors of Metabolism	Tube Feeding Supplies*	Special Feeding Equipment†
USDA: Food Stamps	Certain associated programs may provide general nutrition education that relates to the use of food stamps.	Food stamps may be used to purchase formula that is nutritionally complete.	Food stamps may be used to purchase formula that is nutritionally complete.	N/A	N/A
USDA: National School Lunch and Breakfast Programs	Usually referral is made to a community resource or pediatric clinic for nutrition evaluation.	Must have a diet prescription on file at school for meal modifications, substitutions, and additions, including special formulas; or, specific diet needs must be stated in the IEP or 504 Accommodation Plan.	Must have a diet prescription on file at school for meal modification, substitutions, and additions including special formulas; or, specific diet needs must be stated in the IEP or 504 Accommodation Plan.	N/A	Must be provided by the school if written in the child's IEP; school therapist may also make inexpensive adaptive feeding equipment for children in need.

Table 6.6 (*continued*)

Potential Funding Source	MNT	Pediatric Formula and Tube Feeding Products	Metabolic Formula for the Treatment of Inborn Errors of Metabolism	Tube Feeding Supplies*	Special Feeding Equipment[†]
USDA: WIC	Nutrition evaluation is a required component of the WIC program. For a child with special health care needs, a request should be made for an evaluation by a registered dietitian with special needs training.	Formula provided by prescription; may be limited in selection due to state contract with suppliers; provided as part of food package; quantity limited.	Formula provided by prescription; may be limited selection due to state contract with suppliers; provided as part of food package; quantity is determined by federal regulations.	N/A	N/A

Abbreviations: CSHCN, children with special health care needs; EPSDT, early periodic screening, diagnosis, and treatment; IDEA, Individuals With Disabilities Education Act; IEP, Individualized Education Program; IFSP, Individualized Family Service Plan; MNT, medical nutrition therapy; N/A, not applicable; SCHIP, State Children's Health Insurance Program; SSI, Supplemental Security Income; USDA, United States Department of Agriculture; WIC, Special Supplemental Nutrition Program for Women, Infants, and Children.

*Tubes, pumps, etc.

[†]Special nipples, bottles, spoons, cups, plates, etc.

Clinical Tips

- Partner with families in decision-making about the services and supports for their child. To work together as a team, be open to family views and respectful of the family culture.
- Encourage families to discuss their concerns, questions, and ideas for treatments. Often parents are reluctant to report alternative treatments that they are trying. Hearing the family's questions and concerns is often a first step toward an open discussion to share information about alternative therapies, reinforce helpful and safe strategies, and discourage unsafe practices.
- Remember to encourage grandparents, extended family members, and other caregivers to participate in support and advocacy groups. Sibling groups are also available in certain communities and can provide needed supports for brothers and sisters of CSHCN.
- If parent advocates disagree with clinic or service recommendations, consider involving family specialists from a University Center for Excellence in Developmental Disabilities (UCEDD, formerly university affiliated programs) or a local advisory board, which has parent members. Having active parent participation usually benefits the services the child receives.

Box 6.4   Useful Web Sites

- Title V, CSHCN Program: http://www.mchb.hrsa.gov/programs/default. htm
- US Department of Agriculture (National School Breakfast and Lunch Programs; the Special Supplemental Nutrition Program for Women, Infants, and Children; and Food Stamps Program): http://www.fns. usda.gov/fns
- Individuals with Disabilities Education Act (IDEA), including early intervention and special education:
  - http://www.ed.gov/offices/OSERS/IDEA/regs.html
  - http://nectac.org/partc/partc.asp#overview
  - http://www.fape.org/idea/index.htm
- Medicaid: http://cms.hhs.gov/medicaid
- State Children's Health Insurance Program (SCHIP):
  - http://www.cms.hhs.gov/schip/default.asp
  - http://www.aap.org/advocacy/schiprep.htm
- Supplemental Security Income (SSI): http://www.ssa.gov/pubs/10026. html
- Indian Health Services: http://www.ihs.gov

Case Examples

Example 1

Patient
A 22-month-old girl who was born prematurely and is new to the community.

Problem
Toddler with growth failure requiring special pediatric formula.

Findings
MG was born 2 months premature with bronchopulmonary dysplasia (BPD). Her chronological age is 22 months and her corrected age is 20 months. She has been drinking an infant formula, which is concentrated to provide 24 kcal per ounce, and she consumes approximately 26 oz per day from a bottle. Her mother feeds her three meals of soft table foods and some stage 2 meats. Over the last 6 months, MG has lost 2 lb and her length is stable. She is the only child in a low-income family that is new to the community and has few resources. She is enrolled in an early intervention program because of documented delays in the areas of speech and fine- and gross-motor skills. MG will receive weekly home-based therapy services. The staff is concerned with her lack of growth and recognizes the need for a nutrition evaluation, but a dietetics professional is not a part of their program.

Recommendations
- Refer to Medicaid Program and Title V/CSHCN Program for medical services.
- Refer to WIC program for nutrition services and a specialized food package. If a more in-depth nutrition assessment is needed, the Title V/CSHCN Program may have a dietetics professional on staff or a referral network to complete a nutrition evaluation.
- Develop a plan, monitor progress, and make other appropriate referrals.
- Recommend a complete commercial pediatric formula that provides 30 kcal per ounce as part of the WIC food package. Obtain a prescription for the formula from the primary care physician.
- Request care coordination from the early intervention program to assist the family in coordinating appointments.
- Consult with the WIC or CSHCN Program dietetics professional or nutrition consultant to develop nutrition goals/outcomes and objectives for the IFSP.

Rationale

A variety of resources are available for low-income CSHCN. Early intervention programs provide care coordination for families and can assist with the referral process as well. All programs need to be coordinated to provide continuity of care. The IFSP is an excellent tool to assist families and providers to target goals for a child and to monitor progress. The pediatric nutrition formula will provide increased energy and protein intake without increasing the volume of intake.

Example 2

Patient

An 8-year-old boy with spina bifida and learning disabilities.

Problem

Overweight child who receives special education services and requires diet modifications and new equipment.

Findings

GM is enrolled in the second grade and receives special education services. He has gained 10 lb in the last 6 months, has short stature, and has outgrown his wheelchair. GM participates in the school breakfast and lunch programs. He receives care from a dietetics professional in the regional spina bifida specialty clinic and has Medicaid benefits.

Recommendations

- Design a low-energy diet for weight maintenance and continued linear growth with input from the child and family. Discuss this diet plan with the dietetics professional in the spina bifida clinic.
- Contact the primary care provider to obtain a diet prescription for the school. Discuss plans for the diet with the family and school nutrition program manager. Recommend that the IEP include goals regarding dietary modifications and increased activity level through an adaptive physical education program.
- Refer to physical therapy for evaluation of GM's wheelchair and for processing of paperwork for wheelchair revisions through Medicaid.
- Follow-up in 1 month to monitor progress and adjust the plan as needed.

Rationale

The goal of weight maintenance is appropriate for a growing school-age child. Children with spina bifida usually have a low metabolic rate and need calorie-controlled diets to prevent obesity. Their diets must be planned so that the energy restrictions do not interfere with linear growth. For the best outcome, the meal modifications and activity schedule should be coordinated between the home and school. The IEP is a planning tool to facilitate a coordinated plan. Specialty clinics provide comprehensive care for CSHCN. Some clinics have dietetics professionals on staff, and others may make referrals for nutrition services.

Example 3

Patient
A 1-month-old infant girl who has phenylketonuria (PKU).

Problem
Infant with inborn error of metabolism requires a special metabolic formula and family's managed care plan will not pay for the product.

Findings
ML was diagnosed with PKU shortly after birth through a newborn screening program. Her family's income is more than the income level for Medicaid and WIC services. ML was initially evaluated through the state metabolic treatment program, which is located 1 hour away from her home. She receives follow-up and routine medical exams from her primary care physician through a managed care plan in her community.

Recommendations
- Contact the pharmaceutical company for an initial emergency supply of the formula until other arrangements can be made.
- Enroll family in the state metabolic treatment program through the Title V Program, state health department, which coordinates treatment, medical nutrition therapy by a dietetics professional, and assistance with obtaining the formula.

Rationale
The metabolic formula is necessary to control phenylalanine levels and prevent mental retardation and other medical complications. In many states the metabolic treatment program will provide assistance for families through a sliding fee scale based on family income. The treatment program can provide periodic evaluations and consultations with the local physician. This program is available through the Title V Program in the state health department.

Example 4

Patient
A 7-year-old girl with cystic fibrosis (CF).

Problem
Child with a chronic disease requiring a special diet and support services at school.

Findings
KT is underweight and has lost 4 lb in the past 2 months. She is hungry constantly and eats well at school. KT participates in the school breakfast and lunch programs. She complains about stomach cramps and uses the bathroom frequently. She is self-conscious about taking her enzymes and will often neglect to take them at school. KT is followed by a medical team through a cystic fibrosis center, a specialty clinic at the university medical center. The CF dietetics professional and the medical team reevaluated her and developed the following recommendations.

Recommendations
- Reinforce the need for enzyme replacement therapy before and during intake of meals and snacks.
- Design a meal plan with KT and her family that includes three high-calorie meals and two snacks daily.
- Have parents request a 504 Accommodation Plan that includes a high-calorie diet, scheduled snacks, and monitoring of KT's intake of enzymes. This will reinforce her treatment program at school as well as at home.
- Provide a diet prescription for a high-calorie diet and scheduled snacks at school. Coordinate the plan with the school nutrition program manager.
- Consider counseling for KT to help her with her feelings of self-consciousness.

Rationale
Individuals with CF have insufficient levels of pancreatic enzymes to digest and absorb most fats, proteins, and some carbohydrates. Enzyme replacement therapy is necessary to prevent malabsorption. Children with CF require increased energy intake for their age to meet their high metabolic needs and to support growth. The 504 Plan is the appropriate tool for securing health-related services for students with chronic conditions who are not served in special education

programs. Parents and school personnel contribute to the success of the treatment plan.

References

1. WIC Program, USDA Food and Nutrition Services. Available at: http://www. fns.usda.gov/wic. Accessed July 16, 2003.
2. *Accommodating Children with Special Dietary Needs in School Nutrition Programs: Guidance for School Food Service Staff.* Alexandria, Va: US Department of Agriculture, Food and Nutrition Service; 2001.
3. Medlen JEG. *The Down Syndrome Nutrition Handbook: A Guide to Promoting Healthy Lifestyles.* Bethesda, Md: Woodbine House; 2003.
4. *CARE: Special Nutrition for Kids.* Revised ed. Montgomery, Ala: Alabama State Department of Education, Child Nutrition Programs; 1995.
5. Horsley JW, Allen ER, Daniel PW. *Nutrition Management of School Age Children With Special Needs: A Resource Manual for School Personnel, Families, and Health Professionals.* 2nd ed. Richmond, Va: Virginia Department of Education and Virginia Department of Health; 1996.
6. *Meeting Their Needs: Training Manual for Child Nutrition Program Personnel Serving CSHCN.* Atlanta, Ga: US Department of Agriculture, Food and Nutrition Services, Southeast Regional Office; Birmingham, Ala: University of Alabama at Birmingham, Department of Nutrition Sciences and Sparks Clinics; 1993.
7. Horsley JW, Shockey, WL. Nutrition management for children with special food and nutrition needs. In: Martin J, Conklin MT, eds. *Managing Child Nutrition Programs: Leadership for Excellence.* Gaithersburg, Md: Aspen Publishers; 1999:363–387.

Resources

Books, Manuals, Modules, and Newsletters

Special Health Care Needs

CARE: Special Nutrition for Kids. Department of Education, State of Alabama; 1993.
A manual and instructional videotape for training Child Nutrition program managers about planning and preparing meals for children with special needs.
http://www.olemiss.edu/depts/nfsmi/index.html

The Down Syndrome Nutrition Handbook—A Guide to Promoting Healthy Lifestyles, by JG Medlin. Woodbine House; 2002.
A 430-page handbook for families, educators, and health professionals; covers all life stages.
http://www.woodbinehouse.com

Feeding and Nutrition for the Child with Special Needs: Handouts for Parents, by MD Klein and T Delaney. Therapy Skill Builders; 1994.
A 600-page manual of reproducible handouts on nutrition and feeding issues. Topics include nutrition guidelines, breast and bottle-feeding, introducing food from a spoon, independent feeding, oral-motor treatment strategies, tube feeding, and family mealtime.
http://www.harcourtassessment.com or 800/228-0752

Feeding and Swallowing Disorders in Infancy: Assessment and Management, by LS Wolf and RP Glass. 1992.
Addresses the diagnosis, evaluation, treatment, and follow-up of infants with varying types of feeding dysfunction.
http://www.harcourtassessment.com or 800/228-0752

Interdisciplinary Clinical Assessment of Young Children with Developmental Disabilities, edited by MJ Guralnick. Brookes Publishing Co; 2000.
Includes focus on interdisciplinary process, specific discipline assessments (including nutrition assessment), and interdisciplinary assessment case studies of children with a variety of diagnoses.
http://www.brookespublishing.com

Nutritional Care for High-Risk Newborns, revised 3rd ed. S Groh-Wargo et al. Precept Press; 2000.
> http://www.bonus-books.com

NUTRITION FOCUS for Children with Special Health Care Needs.
> Newsletter published six times annually. Each newsletter focuses on a specific disorder or condition and includes practical strategies and resources for health care professionals.
> http://depts.washington.edu/chdd/ucedd/CO/co_NutriFocus.html

Nutrition Interventions for Children with Special Health Care Needs, by M Nardella et al. Washington State Department of Health; 2002.
> This publication includes 3 sections: determination of nutritional status, problem-based nutrition interventions, and condition-specific nutrition interventions. Available to be downloaded.
> http://depts.washington.edu/cshcnnut/wa_publications.html

Nutrition for Children with Special Health Care Needs, by B Ogata et al. Pacific West MCH Distance Learning Network; 2002.
> Web-based modules that address nutrition assessment of children with special needs and developing effective interventions. Also available on CD-ROM.
> http://depts.washington.edu/pwdlearn

Nutrition Manual for At-Risk Infants and Toddlers, by JH Cox. Precept Press; 1997.
> Provides nutrition information to dietitians, nurses, and physicians to facilitate integration and coordination of services for high-risk infants and toddlers.
> http://www.bonus-books.com

Nutrition Strategies for Children with Special Needs. UAP Center for Child Development and Developmental Disabilities, Children's Hospital Los Angeles; 1999.
> This manual includes nutrition screening forms in English and Spanish, food guidelines for children ages birth to 18 years, 11 sections on specific nutrition concerns, discussion of nutrition issues associated with three specific conditions.
> 323/669-5948

Pediatric Nutrition in Chronic Diseases and Developmental Disorders, by SW Ekvall. Oxford University Press; 1993.
> A review of growth and nutrition for children with chronic diseases and developmental disabilities. Attention is given to assessment of nutritional status and to condition-specific issues.
> http://www.oup.com/us

Pre-Feeding Skills: A Comprehensive Resource for Feeding Development, 2nd ed, by S Morris and M Klein. Therapy Skill Builders; 2000.

A practical manual for feeding assessment and intervention.
http://www.harcourtassessment.com or 800/228-0752

Project Chance, A Guide to Feeding Young Children with Special Needs. Arizona
Department of Health Services, Office of Nutrition Services; 1995.
>Designed to assist early childhood program staff and other caregivers in feeding and
>nourishing children with special needs. Provides general information plus practical
>tips on specific foods to offer.
> http://www.hs.state.az.us/phs/ocshcn/publications/prochance. htm

Project SPOON: Special Program of Oral Nutrition for Children with Special Needs, by
A Tluczek and S Sondel. 1991.
>Report of a 3-year pilot project using a multidisciplinary model to serve parents of
>infants and children with chronic medical conditions. Available from the HRSA
>Information Center, Item Code: MCHE016.
>http://www.ask.hrsa.gov

General Pediatric Nutrition

Bright Futures in Practice: Nutrition, 2nd ed, by D Sofka and M Story. National Center
for Education in Maternal and Child Health; 2002.
>These supervision guidelines emphasize prevention and early recognition of nutri-
>tion concerns for infancy through adolescence. Also available online.
>http://www.brightfutures.org/nutrition

Handbook of Pediatric Nutrition, 2nd ed, by PQ Samour et al. Aspen Publishers, Inc;
1999.
>Includes nutrition information about infants, toddlers, preteens, and adolescents
>and recommendations for nutrition for specific conditions and disorders (revision
>is in press; to be published by Jones and Bartlett Publishers).
>http://www.jbpub.com

Nutrition in Infancy and Childhood, 6th ed, by CM Trahms and PL Pipes. McGraw-Hill;
1997.
>Nutrition information related to growth and development. Addresses the many fac-
>tors that affect and are affected by nutritional status, including development, envi-
>ronment, behavior, and disease.
>http://www.mhhe.com/catalogs/sem/nutrition

Pediatric Manual of Clinical Dietetics, 2nd ed, edited by N Nevin-Folino. American
Dietetic Association; 2003.
>The manual presents guidelines for nutrition assessment and care for a general pedi-
>atric population, as well as for a variety of specific conditions.
>http://www.eatright.org/catalog

Pediatric Nutrition Handbook, 5th ed. American Academy of Pediatrics; 2004.
>   A reference on the nutritional requirements and the effects of nutrition on the health of infants, children, adolescents, and young adults.
>   http://www.aap.org/bookstore

Useful Internet Web sites

Nutrition-Related Web sites

Assuring Pediatric Nutrition in the Community
>   General guidelines, frequently asked questions, resources, continuing education, and training opportunities.
>   http://depts.washington.edu/nutrpeds

CDC Growth Charts
>   Information about and downloadable copies of the 2000 CDC Growth Charts; the site also includes training materials.
>   http://www.cdc.gov/growthcharts
>   Training materials available at: http://depts.washington.edu/growth

Dietary Reference Intakes
>   Downloadable copies of all DRI reports by the Institute of Medicine, National Academy Press.
>   http://www.nap.edu

Gaining and Growing
>   Focus on nutrition follow-up of premature infants in the community.
>   https://staff.washington.edu/growing

Nutrition Services for Children with Special Health Care Needs in Washington State
>   Information for health care providers and families (general and Washington State), including links to reimbursement reports and other resources.
>   http://depts.washington.edu/cshcnnut

US Department of Agriculture
>   Includes the National School Breakfast and Lunch Programs, the Supplemental Nutrition Program for Women, Infants, and Children [WIC], and Food Stamps Program.
>   http://www.fns.usda.gov/fns

For Dietetics Professionals

Dietetics in Developmental and Psychiatric Disorders
>   A dietetic practice group of the American Dietetic Association.
>   http://www.ddpd.org

Pediatric Nutrition Practice Group
>A dietetic practice group of the American Dietetic Association.
>http://www.pediatricnutrition.org

Web sites Related to Medical, Educational, Financial, and Supportive Services

American Association on Mental Retardation
>Professional association promoting policies, research, effective practices, and universal human rights for people with intellectual disabilities.
>http://www.aamr.org

Individuals with Disabilities Education Act (IDEA)
>Includes early intervention and special education.
>http://www.ed.gov/offices/OSERS/IDEA/regs.html
>http://nectac.org/partc/partc.asp#overview
>http://www.fape.org/idea/index.htm

Exceptional Parent Magazine
>Information, support, ideas, and outreach for parents and families of children with disabilities and the professionals who work with them.
>http://www.eparent.com

Family Village
>A global community that integrates information, resources, and communication opportunities on the Internet for persons with cognitive and other disabilities, their families, and service providers.
>http://www.familyvillage.wisc.edu

Family Voices
>Partnering with professionals and families to advocate for health care services that are family-centered, community-based, comprehensive, coordinated, and culturally competent.
>http://www.familyvoices.org

Federal Interagency Coordinating Council
>Established by IDEA legislation serving young children with disabilities; provides links to state interagency coordinating councils.
>http://www.fed-icc.org

Federation for Children with Special Needs
>Massachusetts-based center for parents and parent organizations working on behalf of children with special needs and their families.
>http://www.fcsn.org

Genetic Alliance
Support, education, and advocacy for those living with genetic conditions.
http://www.geneticalliance.org

Indian Health Services, US Department of Health and Human Services
http://www.ihs.gov

Maternal and Child Health Bureau, Health Resources and Services Administration,
US Department of Health and Human Services, Title V programs and Children with Special Health Care Needs Program
http://www.mchb.hrsa.gov/programs/default.htm

Medicaid Program, Centers for Medicare and Medicaid Services, US Department of Health and Human Services
http://cms.hhs.gov/medicaid

National Down Syndrome Society
A comprehensive resource for Down syndrome.
http://www.ndss.org

The National Information Center for Children and Youth with Disabilities
Targeted mainly toward educational programs.
http://www.NICHCY.org

National Organization for Rare Diseases (NORD)
http://www.rarediseases.org

State Children's Health Insurance Program (SCHIP)
http://www.cms.hhs.gov/schip/default.asp
http://www.aap.org/advocacy/schiprep.htm

Supplemental Security Income (SSI), Social Security Administration
http://www.ssa.gov/pubs/10026.html

Glossary

504 Accommodation Plan: Planning document used in schools for children who require health-related services (including modified meals), but who are not enrolled in a special education program; mandated by the Rehabilitation Act of 1973.

achondroplasia: An inherited congenital disorder that is characterized by short stature, short limbs, normal trunk, and specific head/face features (large head, prominent forehead, low nasal bridge).

ADA. *See* Americans with Disabilities Act of 1990 (ADA).

adequate intake (AI): A recommended intake value based on observed or experimentally determined approximations or estimates of nutrient intake by a group (or groups) of healthy people that are assumed to be adequate; used when an RDA cannot be determined.

ADHD. *See* Attention deficit hyperactivity disorder (ADHD).

AGA: Appropriate for gestational age; includes consideration for degree of prematurity.

AI. *See* adequate intake (AI).

Americans with Disabilities Act of 1990 (ADA): federal legislation enacted to protect persons with disabilities from discrimination.

anal stenosis: A condition in which the anus is narrowed.

anthropometric: Pertaining to the science of measuring the body, including height, length, weight, and the size of other body parts.

anticonvulsant: Medications used to prevent or control the occurrence or severity of seizures; medication-nutrient interactions can affect metabolism of vitamins D, B-6, B-12, folic acid, and carnitine.

apnea: Cessation of breathing for a time; a sign of respiratory distress of multifactorial etiology, including prematurity and feeding problems in children with special health care needs.

arm span: The distance between a child's extended right and left middle fingers, measured across the back; sometimes used to estimate height.

ASD. *See under* autism.

aspiration: The drawing or sucking in of foreign material into the lungs, including food, liquid, or stomach contents; clinically significant aspiration requires consideration of non-oral feeding and/or surgery to protect the airway.

ataxia: Imbalance or lack of coordination of voluntary and involuntary movements; seen in neurological disorders (eg, cerebral palsy).

athetoid/athetosis: Condition of ceaseless, involuntary muscle movements; a form of cerebral palsy; can result in increased energy needs.

attention deficit hyperactivity disorder (ADHD): A neurological disorder that results in excessive activity (hyperactivity), impulsivity, and difficulties with focusing attention.

autism: A type of pervasive developmental disorder (PDD) that includes communication problems, ritualistic behaviors, and inappropriate social interactions; part of autism spectrum disorder (ASD).

BMI. *See* body mass index.

body mass index (BMI): An indicator of weight and height proportionality; used in nutrition screening (BMI in 85th to 95th percentile indicates at risk for overweight; BMI > 95th percentile indicates obesity; BMI < 5th percentile indicates underweight); BMI = weight (kg)/height (m)^2.

bolus: Term used in enteral nutrition support to indicate a feeding administered at one time, usually by gastrostomy or nasogastric tube.

BPD. *See* bronchopulmonary dysplasia (BPD).

bronchopulmonary dysplasia (BPD): A chronic lung disorder; most commonly seen in children born prematurely, with low birth weight, or requiring prolonged mechanical ventilation; nutritional consequences can include feeding difficulties, slow growth, and increased energy needs.

cerebral palsy (CP): A nonprogressive motor nerve disorder of the central nervous system; results in muscle coordination difficulties; different parts of the body are affected: hemiplegia affects only the right or left side, diplegia primarily affects the legs, and quadriplegia affects the whole body; movements may be described as spastic (increased tone) or dystonia (slow, rhythmic, twisting), athetoid (involuntary writhing movements), or ataxic (unbalanced jerky movements).

CF. *See* cystic fibrosis.

CHAMPUS. *See* TRICARE.

Children With Special Health Care Needs (CSHCN) program: Federal- (Title V) and state-funded program located in state health departments; promotes and coordinates services for children who have serious physical, behavioral, or emotional conditions that require health and related services beyond those generally required by children.

cleft lip and cleft palate: Conditions occurring when tissues that usually form the lip or the roof of the mouth fail to grow together, creating a gap in the lip or a hole in the roof of the mouth; may be an isolated condition or may be associated with other syndromes; the cleft lip is usually repaired at approximately 3 months of age; the cleft palate is usually repaired at approximately 1 year of age.

CNS: Central nervous system.

congenital heart disease: A cardiac problem that is present at birth, involving one or more defects in the heart, the heart's valves, the veins leading to the heart or the connections among these various parts of the body; usually repaired by surgery early in life.

corrected age: Age from birth, corrected for prematurity; 40 weeks minus gestational age at birth (eg, an infant born at 30 weeks' gestation has a corrected age of 2 weeks at 12 weeks after birth).

CP. *See* cerebral palsy.

crown-rump length: Length between a child's head and buttocks; sometimes used as an estimator of length.

CSHCN: Children with special health care needs. *See also* Children With Special Health Care Needs (CSHCN) program.

cystic fibrosis (CF): An inherited disorder of the endocrine glands, primarily the pancreas, pulmonary system, and sweat glands, characterized by abnormally thick luminal secretions.

diaphragmatic hernia: Protrusion of part of the stomach upwards through an abnormal opening between the thoracic and abdominal cavities; associated with respiratory, cardiac, and gastrointestinal problems.

dietary reference intakes (DRIs): Generic term for a set of nutrient reference values; includes estimated average requirement (EAR), recommended dietary allowance (RDA), adequate intake (AI), tolerable upper intake level (UL), and estimated energy requirement (EER).

Down syndrome: Trisomy 21; a genetic disorder in which the individual has an extra 21st chromosome; characterized by short stature, low muscle tone, cardiac and gastrointestinal problems, cognitive delay, and distinct facial appearance.

DRI. *See* dietary reference intakes (DRIs).

dysphagia: Difficulty in swallowing.

EAR. *See* estimated average requirement (EAR).

Early Head Start: Expansion of the Head Start program to serve low-income pregnant women, infants, and children to age 3 years; program components include education; social services; meals and snacks; health, nutrition, and dental screening and education.

early intervention services: Community-based, comprehensive therapeutic and educational services for infants and children up to 3 years of age with developmental delays; established by Part H of the federal Individuals With Disabilities Education Act (IDEA) of 1986 (now Part C of IDEA, 1997).

Early Periodic Screening, Diagnosis, and Treatment (EPSDT): Program within Medicaid for people younger than 22 years of age; provides medical and dental services; can often provide nutrition-related specialty services, depending on state restrictions.

EER. *See* estimated energy requirement (EER).

encopresis: Fecal incontinence not due to organic defect or illness.

EPSDT. *See* Early Periodic Screening, Diagnosis, and Treatment (EPSDT).

estimated average requirement (EAR): A daily nutrient intake value that is estimated to meet the requirement for half of the healthy individuals in a life state and gender group.

Estimated Energy Requirement (EER): DRI for energy; calculated using PAL.

fundoplication: Surgical procedure that involves mobilizing the lower end of the esophagus and wrapping the fundus of the stomach around it; indicated by diminished function of lower esophageal sphincter or severe/chronic gastroesophageal reflux disease (GERD); sometimes done when placing a gastrostomy tube.

gag reflex: A normal reflex triggered by touching the soft palate or back of the throat, which raises the palate, retracts the tongue, and contracts the throat muscles; protects the airway from a bolus of food or liquid.

gastroesophageal reflux disease (GERD): Regurgitation of stomach contents upward through the lower esophageal sphincter into the esophagus, where they can be aspirated; results in uncomfortable, burning sensation; common cause of feeding and eating problems in infants and children with neuromuscular disabilities.

gastroschisis: A birth defect of incomplete closure of the abdominal wall.

gastrostomy tube: A feeding tube surgically placed through an opening from the abdomen to the stomach; tubes can also be placed endoscopically.

GERD. *See* gastroesophageal reflux disease (GERD).

GI: Gastrointestinal.

glycogen storage diseases: Caused by deficiencies of enzymes that regulate the synthesis or degradation of glycogen; hypoglycemia can be life-threatening; treatment can include nocturnal drip feedings of a carbohydrate-containing solution, or raw cornstarch therapy.

granulation tissue: Connective tissue that forms on the surface of a wound, ulcer, or inflamed tissue surface.

Head Start: Federally funded preschool program for children ages 3 to 5 years from low-income families; includes children with special needs; program components include parent education, meals and snacks, and health, nutrition, and dental screening and education.

health maintenance organization (HMO): A type of managed care.

height-age equivalent: Age at which current length or height would fall at the 50th percentile on the length-for-age or height-for-age growth chart.

Hirschsprung's disease: Congenital absence of nerves in the smooth muscle wall of the colon, resulting in buildup of feces and widening of the bowel (megacolon).

HMO. *See* health maintenance organization (HMO).

hydrocephalus: A congenital or acquired condition with accumulation of cerebrospinal fluid within the skull; characterized by enlarged head, prominent forehead, mental deterioration, and seizures.

hypersensitivity: Abnormal sensitivity; exaggerated response by the body to a stimulus, such as touch, taste, or smell; in feeding problems, hypersensitivity includes adverse reaction or refusal to have mouth touched or teeth brushed, gagging or negative reaction to food in mouth, and tactile defensiveness.

hypertonia: Increased muscle tone; facial hypertonia may result in oral-motor feeding difficulties such as bite reflexes and retracted upper lip.

hypotonia: Diminished muscle tone; can result in poor suck and feeding difficulties.

IBW. *See* ideal body weight (IBW).

ICC. *See* Interagency Coordinating Council (ICC).

IDEA. *See* Individual With Disabilities Education Act of 1997 (IDEA).

ideal body weight (IBW): Weight at 50th percentile for current age.

IEP. *See* Individualized Education Program (IEP).

IFSP. *See* Individualized Family Service Plan (IFSP).

Indian Health Services: Federal program to provide health services to Native Americans.

Individualized Education Program (IEP): Planning document required annually for special education services in public schools serving children older than 3 years; outlines specific goals, activities, and timelines.

Individualized Family Service Plan (IFSP): Planning document required for services for children from birth to 3 years of age enrolled in early intervention services; includes specific goals, activities, and timelines.

Individual With Disabilities Education Act of 1997 (IDEA): Federal education legislation; Part C includes early intervention services.

Interagency Coordinating Council (ICC): Each state providing early intervention services under IDEA (Part C) has an ICC located in the state government.

IVH: Intraventricular hemorrhage; graded 1 (mild) to 4 (major); in premature infants, may be associated with subsequent neurological damage and developmental disability.

jaw grading: Ability to control the degree of movement of the lower jaw; a feeding skill important in accepting food from a spoon and in biting and chewing.

jaw retraction: Involuntary movement of the jaw backward, making it difficult to open the mouth voluntarily; a common oral-motor feeding problem that interferes with the ability to handle food textures.

low birth weight (LBW): Used to describe a newborn weighing less than 2,500 g (5.5 lb) and less than 38 weeks' gestation.

macrocephaly: Excessively large size of head.

Marfan syndrome: Congenital disorder of the connective tissue characterized by excessive length of the fingers and toes and other deformities.

MCT. *See* medium-chain triglycerides (MCT).

Medicaid: Federal medical assistance program for children from low-income families; often matched by state funds.

medium-chain triglycerides (MCT): Type of fatty acid.

microcephaly: Small head size in relation to age and other growth parameters; may reflect inadequate brain growth; common feature of neurological damage before or immediately after birth.

modified barium swallow: A radiologic study of the oral and pharyngeal cavities to evaluate the swallowing mechanism; foods and liquids are mixed with barium and the feeding is recorded on videotape; also called *videofluoroscopic swallowing study* (VFSS).

munching: Oral-motor feeding developmental stage characterized by up-and-down movement of the jaw; occurs before development of rotary chewing.

myelomeningocele. *See* spina bifida.

myotonic dystrophy: An inherited autosomal dominant neuromuscular disorder that occurs in adults; characterized by progressive muscle weakness, wasting, and mytonia.

nasogastric feeding: A form of enteral nutrition support; tube runs from nose into stomach; usually used temporarily (eg, < 3 months).

National School Breakfast and Lunch Program: School program in which children receive a balanced morning and midday meal; sponsored by the USDA's Child Nutrition Program.

Nellhaus chart: Standard reference for head circumference in infants and children from birth to age 18 years.

NICU: Neonatal intensive care unit.

Noonan syndrome: A disorder marked by short stature, webbing of the neck, mental retardation, and craniofacial features (wide mouth, protruding upper lip).

obstipation: Constipation resulting in accumulation of feces with development of colon distention; leads to fecal impaction.

obstructive lesions: Conditions where a normal body passage is partly or completely obstructed; examples of those affecting eating and nutrition include pyloric stenosis, tracheoesophageal fistula, duodenal atresia.

oral rehydration therapy (ORT): Slow oral administration of glucose, sodium, potassium, and chloride to replace fluid and electrolyte losses and correct extracellular fluid volume after mild or severe dehydration.

ORT. *See* oral rehydration therapy (ORT).

PAL. *See* physical activity level (PAL).

palmar grasp: Hand movement in which the palm rather than the fingertips make contact with an object for grasping; developmental stage that is an important precursor to self-feeding.

PDD: pervasive developmental disorder.

phasic bite reflex: Opening and closing of the jaw that occurs when the gums and teeth are stimulated.

phenylketonuria (PKU): An amino acid disorder inherited as an autosomal recessive; marked by the deficiency of the enzyme that converts phenylalanine to tyrosine; accumulation of phenylalanine in the blood can lead to mental retardation and other neurological problems; identified in newborn screening; treatment includes a special diet with medical foods.

physical activity level (PAL): Coefficient used to determine estimated energy requirements (EER).

Pierre-Robin syndrome: Disorder characterized by small lower jaw and abnormal smallness of the tongue; often with cleft palate or with other malformations; results in respiratory and feeding problems; also called *Robin sequence.*

pincer grasp: Refined, mature hand movement in which the thumb and index finger are used to grasp a small object; a developmental stage that is an important skill in self-feeding.

PKU. *See* phenylketonuria (PKU).

positioning: Physical management of posture and body alignment to support daily living skills such as standing and eating.

post-ictal: Following a seizure.

Prader-Willi syndrome: Genetic disorder of chromosome 15 marked by hypotonia, short stature, hyperphagia, and developmental disabilities; characterized by poor feeding in infancy, and when not carefully managed, excessive weight gain in children and adults.

preterm: Term used to describe an infant who is born prematurely at less than 38 weeks' gestation.

RDA. *See* recommended dietary allowance (RDA).

recognized medical authority: Term in federal regulations pertaining to Child Nutrition Programs that refers to a physician, physician's assistant, registered nurse, nurse practitioner, registered dietitian, or other specialist identified by the state agency (eg, Department of Education).

recommended dietary allowance (RDA): The intake that meets the nutrient need of almost all (97%-98%) of individuals in a group.

Rett syndrome: A neurological disorder of females, marked by progressive neurological deterioration, seizures, and cognitive impairment.

Robin sequence. *See* Pierre-Robin syndrome.

rooting reflex: Newborn reflex in which the infant turns his head toward the hand or nipple stroking his cheek, and initiates sucking.

rotary chewing: Movement of jaw side-to-side and up-and-down to grind and mash food; a mature developmental feeding stage in which a wide variety of food textures can be handled.

SCHIP. *See* State Children's Health Insurance Program (SCHIP).

scoliosis: Lateral curvature of the vertebral column; associated with some congenital and neurological disorders.

seizure disorder: Involuntary movement or changes in consciousness or behavior brought on by abnormal bursts of electrical activity in the brain; seizures can be classified as general or partial; when seizures occur repeatedly they are diagnosed as epilepsy.

sensory integration (SI) therapy: Techniques, used by some speech-language therapists, occupational therapists, or physical therapists, aimed at helping children sort out and organize their senses, thereby improving hypersensitivities or hyposensitivities and fine-motor skills.

SGA. *See* small for gestational age (SGA).

SI therapy. *See* sensory integration (SI) therapy.

sitting height: Length between a child's head and buttocks; sometimes used as an estimator of height.

small for gestational age (SGA): Birth weight < 10th percentile for age.

spastic: Increased muscle tone and stiffness; descriptor for cerebral palsy.

Special Olympics: An international program of year-round sports training and athletic competition for children and adults with mental retardation.

Special Supplemental Feeding Program for Women, Infants, and Children (WIC): A federal program providing foods, infant formula, and nutrition education to pregnant and breastfeeding women, infants, and children younger than 5 years of age.

spina bifida: A congenital defect in which part of the spinal column fails to close completely during fetal development, resulting in a hernia (containing the spinal cord, the meninges, and cerebral spinal fluid) along the spinal column; higher lesions result in greater limitations in mobility; long-term nutritional risks include overweight, constipation, and reduced energy needs; also called *myelomeningocele.*

SSI. *See* Supplemental Security Income (SSI).

State Children's Health Insurance Program (SCHIP): A federal Medicaid children's health insurance program created in 1997; optional program for states to offer uninsured or underinsured children who generally do not qualify for Medicaid; different names in different states.

static encephalopathy: A general term for a neurological or brain disorder that is stable.

steatorrhea: Excessive amounts of fats in the feces; stool characterized by light color and offensive odor; feces float.

sucking: A more mature up-and-down movement of the tongue and jaw, with negative pressure, to extract liquid from a nipple.

suckling: The earliest intake pattern in infants; the lower jaw and tongue elevate and move back and forth, using pressure on the nipple to extract fluid during feeding; replaced by sucking.

Supplemental Security Income (SSI): Federal- and state-funded program that provides supplemental income to offset expenses for children with disabilities who come from low-income families.

TEE. *See* total energy expenditure.

texture: Consistency of food at the time it is served; generally based on amount of mastication required before swallowing.

tolerable upper intake level (UL): The maximum level of daily nutrient intake that is likely to pose no risk of adverse effects for almost all individuals in the general population; unless otherwise specified, the UL represents total intake from food, water, and supplements; ULs are not established for vitamin K, riboflavin, vitamin B-12, pantothenic acid, biotin, or carotenoids.

tongue lateralization: Ability to move the tongue voluntarily from side to side from its midline position; developmental stage in feeding that signals the ability to manipulate food inside the mouth.

tongue retraction: Involuntary tongue movement toward the back of the mouth on presentation of food, spoon, or cup; blocks the normal steps to swallowing.

tongue thrust: Forceful protrusion of the tongue, often in response to an oral stimulus, such as a spoon or food; interferes with moving food from the front of the mouth to the back for swallowing.

tonic bite reflex: Involuntary bite reflex with associated tension; the bite is not easily released (eg, appears that child is biting spoon or finger and cannot release it).

total energy expenditure (TEE): The intake that meets the average energy expenditure of individuals at the reference height, weight, and age.

tracheomalacia: Softening of the cartilage rings in the trachea; results in feeding difficulties with risk of apnea and aspiration during eating.

transpyloric feeding: Nutrition support in which a tube extends from the nose through the stomach, past the pyloric valve, into the first part of the small intestine; used primarily when the person is at risk for aspiration of stomach contents.

TRICARE: A health insurance program for families in the US military; formerly called CHAMPUS.

triceps skinfold measure: Measurement of the skin and subcutaneous fat layer around the triceps muscle; used with arm circumference measurement to estimate fat and muscle stores.

Trisomy 21. *See* Down syndrome.

Turner syndrome: Disorder in females from the absence of one X chromosome; marked by short stature, ovarian failure, and cardiac problems.

UL. *See* Tolerable Upper Intake Level (UL).

ventricular septal defect (VSD): Cardiac anomaly that requires medical or surgical treatment; usually requires increased energy needs.

very low birth weight (VLBW): Descriptor of a premature infant who weighs less than 1,500 g (3.5 1b) at birth.

VFSS. *See* videofluoroscopic swallowing study (VFSS).

videofluoroscopic swallowing study (VFSS): a radiologic study of the oral and pharyngeal cavities to evaluate the swallowing mechanism; foods and liquids are mixed with barium and the feeding is recorded on videotape; also called *modified barium swallow study.*

VLBW. *See* very-low-birth-weight (VLBW).

VSD. *See* ventricular septal defect (VSD).

weight-age equivalent: Age at which current weight would fall at the 50th percentile on the weight-for-age growth chart.

WIC. *See* Special Supplemental Feeding Program for Women, Infants, and Children (WIC).

Williams syndrome: A disorder characterized by distinctive facial features (large lips, small eyes, depressed nasal bridge), growth and developmental delays, cardiac defects, and possible hypercalcemia in infancy.

Index

Page numbers with *b* indicates boxes; with *f*, figures; and *t*, tables.